M000107254

Woodstock '69:

Three Days of Peace,

Music, & Medical Care

Woodstock'69:

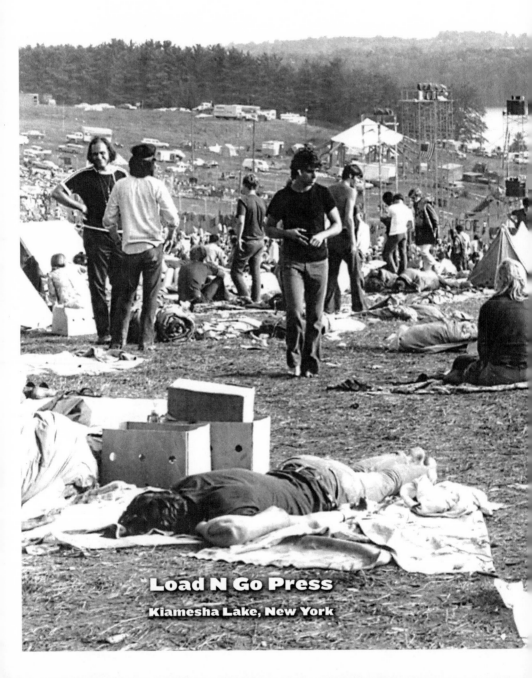

Load N Go Press
Kiamesha Lake, New York

Three Days of Peace, Music, & Medical Care

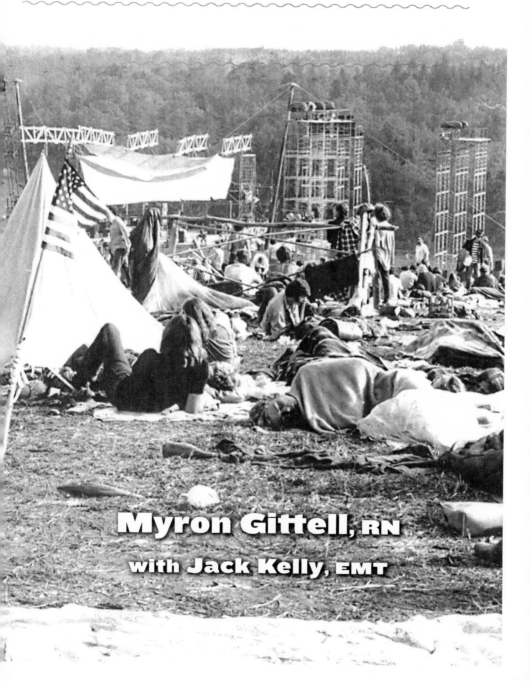

Myron Gittell, RN

with **Jack Kelly,** EMT

Photo credits

Ralph Ackerman © Patricia Ackerman: 72
Paul Gerry, courtesy of the Museum at Bethel Woods: 19, 24, 78, 79, 80
Myron Gittell: *x*
John B. Huggler, Jr.: 25 *(top and bottom)*
Lisa Law: 20, 23, 29, 32, 37, 38-39, 47, 48 *(bottom)*, 54, 59, 74, 93, 109, 118
Barry Z. Levine: 26, 55, 66, 76 *(top and bottom)*
Leslie Teichholz/The Image Works: 34, 45
New York Times: 102
New York State: 77, 87
John Niflot: *ii-iii*, 2 (tickets), 5, 10, 16-17, 106, 110
Tom Miner/The Image Works: 57
Howard Perlman: 98
Walter Saunders: 156
Middletown *Times Herald Record*: 14, 33, 35, 48 *(top)*, 60, 75, 85, 95, 99, 113
Port Jervis *Union Gazette*: 100
Barron Wallman: 44, 63, 71, 73, 90, 92

Published by Load N Go Press
Box 175 Kiamesha Lake, New York 12751
(845)794-3772
myrongit@yahoo.com

Printed in the United States of America

ISBN 9780962635731
Library of Congress Control Number: 2009906034

Designed by Joy Taylor (JoyTaylorDesign.com)

**There is always a
little bit of heaven in a disaster area**

—*Wavy Gravy*

Acknowledgments

I APPRECIATE the invaluable assistance of Wade Lawrence and Robin Green of the Museum at Bethel Woods, who are helping to keep alive the memory of Woodstock '69. Paul Gerry's photos from the Museum's Collections were important additions to the book.

William Burns and company of the Sullivan County Historical Society at the Museum in Hurleyville generously shared their time and resources.

I received tremendous assistance from Robert Dadras and the Liberty Museum and Arts Center. Sherry Mohan of the Port Jervis Gazette, and librarians Pat Racine the Middletown Times Herald-Record, Arlene Shaner of the New York Academy of Medicine, Peggy Johansen of the Livingston Manor Free Library, and my favorite librarian, Maryallison Farley at the Catskill Regional Medical Center, all helped guide me toward important sources.

Thanks to my brother Arnold Gittell and Diana Levine for research help and suggestions; to Howard Perlman for telling his story and for his Super 8mm coverage of the Rutherford School.

The local media through Bill James of WSUL, Dan Hust, Ruth Huggler and Suzanne White of the Sullivan County Democrat, and Barbara Bedell from the Middletown Times Herald-Record, helped the community know of my project and my need for sources.

Barbara Smith provided both transcription services and great food. Wray Rominger of Purple Mountain Press helped out with valuable guidance whenever asked.

Many participants spent the time to share valuable memories of the event, including Ruth Aprilante, R.N., Anna Benson, R.N., Gustave Gavis, M.D., Mischa Leshner, Helen Reno, Lisa Law, and Frances Marks, R.N.

For sharing photos from their private collections special thanks to John Niflot, Ruth Huggler and Pat Ackerman.

Thanks again to Lynn Skolnick for manuscript review, Peter Osborne of the Minisink Valley Historical Society for sharing his knowledge of publishing and history and the Town of Cochecton Preservation Society for inviting me to speak about the Festival.

And special thanks to Ian and Barry Cooperstein of the Town of Liberty Volunteer Ambulance Corps, for digging through the Corps' records from forty years back.

Thank heaven, none of our fears were realized.
What happened at Bethel this past weekend was that those
young people together with our local residents turned the
Aquarian Festival into a dramatic victory for the spirit of
peace, good will and human kindness.....

With the aid of Armed Forces helicopters and local volunteers a
potential medical crisis was averted. They deserve the highest
possible commendation, each and every one, for the tireless
and magnificent way in which they handled the situation....

If half a million people at the Aquarian Festival could
turn such adverse conditions, filled with the possibility of
disaster, riot, looting and catastrophe into three days of music
and peace then perhaps there is hope that if we join with them
we can turn those adversities that are the problems of America
today into a hope for a brighter and more peaceful future.

−Max Yasgur
August 18, 1969

Contents

~~~~~~~~

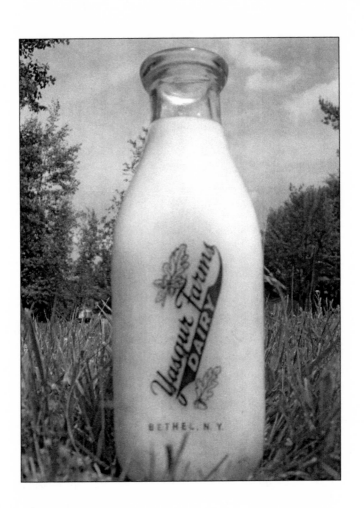

Preface

BACK in the early 1990s, I was attending a Sullivan County Ambulance Association meeting to discuss an upcoming "mock disaster" training exercise. Woodbourne Fire Department First Aid Squad's longtime representative Al Whittaker asked if anyone knew where one of the biggest real medical disasters in America took place? We were stumped until Al told us that it had taken place right in our own backyard.

The 1969 Woodstock Festival, which occurred 12 miles from where I lived and still live, attracted 500,000 attendees, and more than 3,000 of them needed treatment for illness, injury or reactions to street drugs. Those numbers alone make the festival one of the significant disaster scenes in modern America.

As a volunteer Emergency Medical Technician with the Monticello Volunteer Ambulance Corps and a history buff specializing in topics that include the history of emergency medical care and ambulances, I was intrigued by the subject and began collecting information and memories of the historic event from a medical perspective.

Fast-forward to the summer of 2006 when the Liberty Museum, as part of their annual Woodstock coverage, invited me to put together a program on medical care at the 1969 Festival. My interest in telling this fascinating story was rekindled and by digging through contemporary accounts, mining public records, and tapping the memories of participants, I eventually had enough material for a book.

Because the story deserved a readable and dynamic narrative, I collaborated with Jack Kelly, a professional journalist who had written about the history of Emergency Medical Services for *American Heritage Magazine* – and interviewed me in the process.

I have been a medical provider through most of my career, both as an EMT and a registered nurse. Back in 1969, I attended the Woodstock Festival not in any medical capacity, but as a spectator and a Sno-Cone salesman. My friend had a concession on the festival site for the icy treat and was doing a land-office business in what proved to be an early version of "fluid replacement therapy."

I know from firsthand experience that the scene at the Woodstock Festival was, at best, chaotic. Half a million attendees took away half a million memories of the iconic event. From those memories and from the sometimes sketchy records, I have reconstructed the most accurate account that I could of the problems the medical people faced and the ways they handled it. In any case, the numbers only tell part of the story. The compassionate and creative effort by hundreds of volunteers to avert a potential disaster is the story that comes through.

The events described in this book took place in a time now colored by nostalgia. It was an era of idealism, when fresh faces were turned toward the future. Young people in those days often referred to strangers as "brother" and "sister."

Two young men who attended the festival at Yasgur's farm, Raymond Mizsak and Richard Beiler, both teenagers with the prospect of life before them, did not return home. Although their names were never listed among those of the celebrated and famous, they deserve to be remembered. They were our brothers.

Woodstock '69:

Three Days of Peace,

Music, & Medical Care

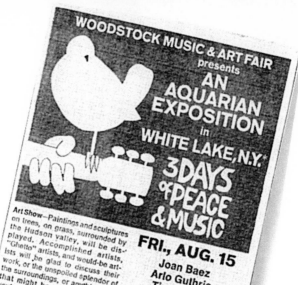

WOODSTOCK MUSIC & ART FAIR
presents
AN AQUARIAN EXPOSITION
in
WHITE LAKE, N.Y.
3 DAYS of PEACE & MUSIC

Art Show—Paintings and sculptures on trees, on grass, surrounded by the Hudson valley, will be displayed. Accomplished artists, "Ghetto" artists, and would-be artists will be glad to discuss their work, or the unspoiled splendor of the surroundings, or anything else that might be on your mind. If you're an artist, and you want to display, write for information.

Crafts Bazaar—If you like creative knickknacks and old junk you'll love roaming around our bazaar. You'll see imaginative leather, ceramic, bead, and silver creations, as well as Zodiac Charts, camp clothes, and worn out shoes.

Work Shops—If you like playing with beads, or improvising on a guitar, or writing poetry, or molding clay, stop by one of our work shops and see what you can give and take.

Food—There will be cokes and hot-dogs and dozens of curious food and fruit combinations to experiment with.

Hundreds of Acres to Roam on—Walk around for three days without seeing a skyscraper or a traffic light. Fly a kite, sun yourself. Cook your own food and breathe the unspoiled air.

Music starts at 4:00 P.M. on Friday, and at 1:00 P.M. on Saturday and Sunday—it'll run for 12 continuous hours, except for a few short breaks to allow the performers to catch their breath.

All programs subject to change without notice
✳White Lake, Town of Bethel (Sullivan County), N.Y.

FRI., AUG. 15

Joan Baez
Arlo Guthrie
Tim Hardin
Richie Havens
Incredible String Band
Ravi Shankar
Sweetwater

SAT., AUG. 16

Keef Hartley
Canned Heat
Creedence Clearwater
Grateful Dead
Janis Joplin
Jefferson Airplane
Mountain
Santana
The Who

SUN., AUG. 17

The Band
Jeff Beck Group
Blood, Sweat and Tears
Joe Cocker
Crosby, Stills and Nash
Jimi Hendrix
Iron Butterfly
The Moody Blues
Johnny Winter

Please Print
☐ Send me information on the WOODSTOCK MUSIC & ART FAIR
Send me ____ tickets for Fri., Aug. 15, at $7.00 each
Send me ____ tickets for Sat., Aug. 16, at $7.00 each
Send me ____ tickets for Sun., Aug. 17, at $7.00 each
Send me ____ 2 day tickets for Fri. & Sat., Aug. 15, 16, at $13.00 each
Send me ____ 2 day tickets for Sat. & Sun., Aug. 16, 17, at $13.00 each
Send me ____ Complete 3 day tickets for Fri., Sat., Sun., Aug. 15, 16, 17, at $18.00 each

Name _____
Address _____
City _____
_____ State _____ Zip _____

Be sure to enclose a self-addressed, stamped envelope with your check or money order (no cash please) payable to:

---

and Art Fair

THREE DAY TICKET

...st 17, 1969
10 A.M.
Aug. 15, 16, 17, 1969

$6.00
$18.00

Good For One Admission Only   NO REFUNDS

80745   80745

Introduction

The Calm Before

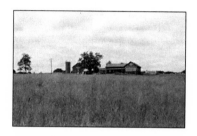

D URING a normal August in the late 1960s, Bethel, New York, was a busy place. The Sullivan County township, about 100 miles northwest of New York City, was located in a region of resort hotels and bungalow colonies known as the "borscht belt." Every summer the region attracted a mostly Jewish clientele from the New York metropolitan area for their holidays.

The hotels—Grossinger's, The Concord, and Kutshers were three of the prominent ones – offered Kosher food and featured entertainers who ranged from Lenny Bruce to Joan Rivers. By 1969, the golden age of the Catskills had passed, but more than 500 hotels and bungalow colonies still operated, swelling the area's population every summer. During the weekend of the Woodstock festival, singer Leslie Uggams, who had been featured on Mitch Miller's *Sing Along With Mitch* television show in the early 1960s, performed at the Concord, and balladeer Julius LaRosa entertained a crowd at the nearby Evans Hotel with his 1950s hit "Eh, Cumpari."

Although the region was often referred to as part of the Catskill Mountains, the terrain was hilly, not rugged – Catskill State Park lay about 30 miles farther north. The rolling hills and abundant lakes of Bethel made for a pleasant setting but the rocky soil restricted agriculture mostly to dairy farming, and many farmers supplemented their income by operating boarding houses on the side.

The residents of Bethel were not country bumpkins; they were used to an annual influx of visitors from the city. Hospital personnel had to prepare every summer for a busy season and facilities were more flexible than those in remoter areas. But July and August *were* the peak of the season, so hospitals and doctors were already busy before the Woodstock hordes arrived.

But they could have had no idea what was about to descend on them as the three-day weekend of August 15, 16, and 17 approached. Earlier rock festivals gave only a hint of the potential for disaster.

One of the first outdoor rock concerts lasting more than one day had taken place in Monterey, California two years earlier. The Monterey International Pop Music Festival in June 1967 had drawn 60,000 fans to a fairground. Some of the same bands that entertained at Woodstock were at Monterey, including the Grateful Dead, Santana, and Jimi Hendrix. The filmmaker D.A. Pennebaker released an influential documentary called *Monterey Pop* in 1968, spawning wide interest in similar extended festivals.

The Monterey Festival took place at the peak of the "Summer of Love," which kicked off the hippie movement and made marijuana and LSD the drugs of choice for young people. The "freakouts" experienced by some users at Monterey gave intimations of a potentially serious drug problem at Woodstock.

Another multiday festival was held at Gulfstream Race Track in Miami, Florida, on May 18 and 19, 1968. It attracted a crowd of more than 100,000 and again featured groups that would appear at Woodstock. One of the producers of the Miami Pop Festival was Michael Lang, the moving force behind the Woodstock event.

Also feeding the dynamic of Woodstock was the "be-in." This type of event was pioneered in January 1967 in Golden Gate Park,

San Francisco. Planned as a protest against the criminalization of LSD, the gathering of about 25,000 people, some of whom were stoned on the drug, generated publicity and inspired similar events touted as "gatherings of the tribe." New York City saw several such events in Central Park from 1967 through 1969. Those be-ins included protests against the unpopular war in Vietnam, then at its height.

There was a built-in contradiction between a "gathering of the tribe" and a commercial music concert. One was a free event with the audience as the principal entertainment and politics as part of the mix. The other was a commercial venture designed for profit. The blending of the two ideas sometimes made for trouble.

In July 1969 the venerable Newport Jazz Festival included a number of popular rock bands, including Sly and the Family Stone and, improbably, Led Zeppelin. The young fans the music attracted, unable to afford local hotels, slept illegally on exclusive Newport beaches. They engaged in a certain amount of unruliness

The Cost of Tickets

The advance-sale cost of tickets to the Woodstock Music and Arts Fair was $7 per day, the equivalent of about $32 in 2009 dollars. The $18 price for the weekend would equal $81 today.

In 1969 a new Chevrolet Impala cost $3,000 (a 2009 model goes for $24,000). Those driving to Woodstock paid 35 cents for a gallon of gas. The minimum wage was $1.60 per hour.

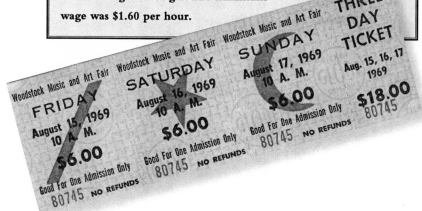

and gate crashing. The attendance of 85,000 broke all records but the young and restless crowd made promoters nervous.

In August, just two weeks before Woodstock, the Atlantic City Pop Music Festival was held at a race track in the New Jersey resort 130 miles south of New York City. The crowd of more than 100,000 pointed to the enormous popularity of such events. Again the lineup of groups overlapped with those that would appear at the Woodstock Festival in Bethel. The event, strictly commercial, was uneventful and quickly forgotten.

The Woodstock Festival had its origins in the idea, originated by Michael Lang and Capitol Records executive Artie Kornfeld, of building a recording studio in Woodstock, NY. The upstate artists' colony had attracted musicians like Bob Dylan, Jimi Hendrix, and Van Morrison, so why not give them a state-of-the-art facility just down the road? To finance the studio, they decided in early 1969 to hold a concert. Maybe they would turn it into a yearly event along the lines of the Newport Festival.

Lang and Kornfeld had by this time connected with two young financiers, John Roberts and Joel Rosenman, who would bankroll Woodstock Ventures, the company that sponsored the festival. They originally had the idea of holding the event in Woodstock itself. The objections of local residents and other factors led the promoters to move the festival to nearby Saugerties. When that offer was withdrawn, they located a 600-acre industrial park in the town of Wallkill on the outskirts of the small city of Middletown, New York, but could not get the town's zoning board to approve.

With barely a month to go, the promoters managed to secure a lease on Max Yasgur's farm in the Town of Bethel in Sullivan County. A carefully planned advertising campaign combined with effective word-of-mouth marketing and the booking of many of the top rock and folk acts of the day, kept interest growing all summer. The rural location now added to the mystique of the event, as most rock festivals had been held at race tracks or fairgrounds. This would be more than just a rock concert -- it would be, as the slogan said, "Three days of Peace and Music . . . An Aquarian Exposition."

The Woodstock Festival would combine elements of both a

concert and a be-in, a commercial entertainment and a gathering of a large and amorphous tribe. As the event swelled in size, the commercial element was partly lost. Promoters declared it a free concert, hoping to recoup their investment from the Warner Brothers movie which was already in the works. The music remained an important, but secondary element to the simple assembly of half a million like-minded people eager for a party.

The size of the crowd and the inadequate planning had the potential to turn the August event into a serious, life-threatening disaster. Yet Woodstock lent its name not only to a generation, but also to an idea of cooperation rather than competition, of love and peace rather than ego and aggression.

One of the critical factors that prevented catastrophe was the improvised effort on the part of hundreds of nurses, doctors and others, some paid, many volunteers, who took over and managed a large-scale medical emergency with determination and dedication. This book tells the story of that hurried, sometimes frenzied, often chaotic, ultimately successful effort to provide health and healing to half a million people.

A Farmer with Soul

As a young man, Max Yasgur had studied real estate at New York University, but he decided to return home to help run his family's dairy farm. He bought more land and by 1969 he ran the largest dairy operation in Sullivan County, milking 650 Guernseys. A large, gaunt 49-year-old with glasses at the time of the festival, Max was already suffering from the heart problem that would kill him four years later.

Yasgur rented out a portion of his farm for the festival and pitched in to help make it a success. Noted as a down-to-earth man of his word, Yasgur hoped that the festival would help close the generation gap.

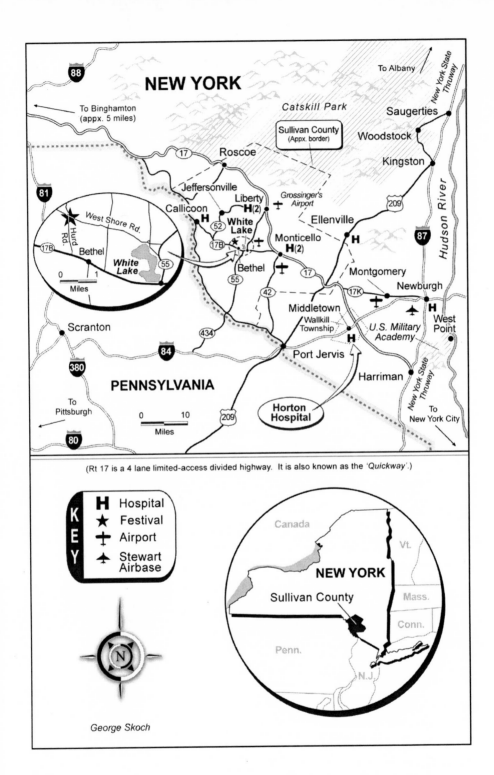

NEW YORK

To Binghamton
(appx. 5 miles)

Catskill Park

Sullivan County
(Appx. border)

Roscoe

To Albany

New York State Thruway

Saugerties

Woodstock

Kingston

Jeffersonville

Liberty **H**(2)

Grossinger's Airport

Callicoon

H

52

White Lake

Ellenville

209

Hudson River

West Shore Rd.

Hurd Rd.

17B

Bethel

White Lake

55

17B

Monticello
H(2)

Montgomery

H

87

0   1

Miles

Bethel

55

17

Newburgh

17K

42

Middletown

Wallkill Township

U.S. Military Academy

West Point

H

Scranton

434

84

380

PENNSYLVANIA

Port Jervis

H

Harriman

New York State Thruway

To
Pittsburgh

0   10

Miles

209

Horton
Hospital

To
New York City

80

(Rt 17 is a 4 lane limited-access divided highway. It is also known as the 'Quickway'.)

**K
E
Y**

H Hospital
★ Festival
✝ Airport
✈ Stewart
Airbase

N

Canada

NEW YORK

Vt.

Sullivan County

Mass.

Conn.

Penn.

N.J.

George Skoch

8

(Opposite) Woodstock Festival site marked with a star, and surrounding area.

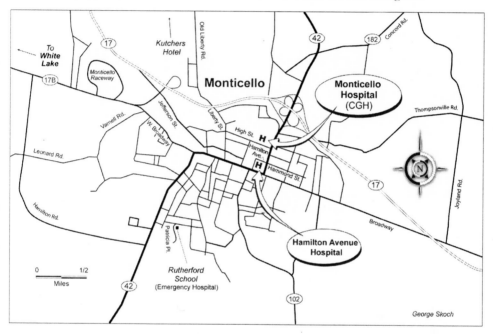

(Above) Greater Monticello

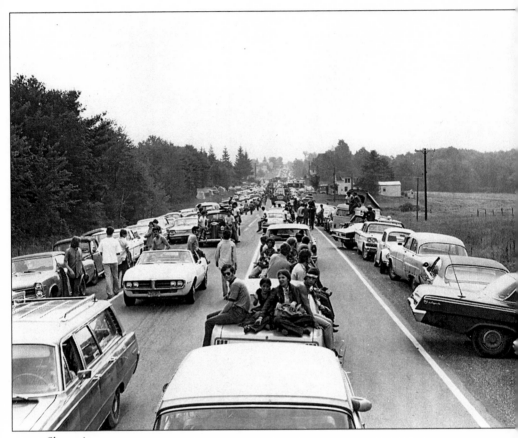

Slow going

1

~~~~~~~~~~~~~~~~~~

The Gathering Storm

W E HAVE the makings of a medical disaster here," said one
volunteer physician.[1]

The planners had envisioned that a crowd of 50,000
would be on hand that August weekend for three days of music, art
and nature in the rolling farmland of Sullivan County, about two
hours from New York City.

But even before it opened, the Woodstock Music and Art Fair
was growing out of all proportion. A mass of people eight times as
large as anticipated was descending on the site. The possibility of a
million human beings trying to crowd onto the remote 600-acre
patch of farmland put the fear of God into those responsible for the
fair-goers' welfare. A rule of thumb predicted that a crowd as big
as the one already gathering would result in as many as 20 deaths.
One of the promoters thought there would be a "holocaust" if they
didn't stop the festival.[2]

Catastrophe was in the air. The previous year had been the most
violent in post-World War II history: Martin Luther King Jr. and
Bobby Kennedy assassinated, colleges torn by strikes and violence, a
"police riot" at the Chicago Democratic convention. It was also the

bloodiest year of the Vietnam war, which had flared up in 1965 and would continue another seven years. In 1968, 17,000 Americans died in Southeast Asia — and the war continued.

Now a multitude of young people were on the march toward a poorly planned event in the middle of nowhere and nobody knew what the consequences would be.

"The wrong vibes, as we used to call it, could have sent that thing into a violent riot," Abbie Hoffman remembered. Hoffman, one of the best-known radical social activists of the era, was worried. "I mean, it could have been five hundred to a thousand dead just from panicking," he said later.[3] Given the crowds, conditions, drug use, and lack of organized security, his concern was not necessarily exaggerated.

In fact the doctor in charge of emergency medical care at Woodstock feared the possibility of "the greatest medical tragedy of our times."[4]

The arriving masses swept away all notions of crowd control at the site. Thousands had already entered the grounds by Thursday, before the fences and gates were completed. To force them out and let in only ticket holders became an impossibility. Even before the scheduled kickoff time of 4:00 p.m. Friday, the event was declared a free concert. In part, the decision was made in order to assure that the movie being made of the festival was not marred by an ugly scene; in part, the numbers of people were simply overwhelming all efforts to maintain order. Crowds flattened the hurricane fences and swarmed onto the site.

That same day, the 346 off-duty New York City police who had been hired as "Peace Reserve Corps" were ordered off the job by Police Commissioner Howard Leary because of a city rule against moonlighting. And while 200 off-duty officers would stay to help out (many of the city cops under assumed names), the security force would be far from adequate for the huge gathering. By Friday morning, notices were being sent out on radio stations for spectators to turn back. The inadequate roads were quickly congealing. Many attendees left their cars and walked, some for a dozen miles. Abandoned cars added to the congestion.

"Anybody who tries to come here is crazy," said Woodstock Ventures security chief Wes Pomeroy. "Sullivan County is a great big parking lot."[5]

There is no question that the Woodstock festival the "Rock Rumble in Rip Van Winkle Country," as one newspaper called it -- was teetering on the brink of disaster.[6] As everyone knows, that disaster never happened. There was no riot, no panic.

The death of two fair-goers was a tragedy, but prompt medical attention saved the lives of others. The care of the sick and injured

---

The Hospitals

Community General Hospital (CGH; now Catskill Regional Medical Center) operated two hospitals near Bethel. The closest, in Monticello, ten miles away, had 94 beds. The one in Liberty, 12 miles distant, had 80 beds. Both prepared as well as they could, calling in personnel and discharging any patients they could beforehand. The crush of patients from the festival soon overwhelmed both facilities. Two smaller private hospitals, Liberty-Loomis in Liberty and Hamilton Avenue Hospital in Monticello, helped relieve overcrowding by handling some of the patients.

Horton Memorial Hospital in Middletown, 35 miles from the site, and St. Luke's Hospital in Newburgh, 58 miles away, were larger facilities with more comprehensive capabilties. Both took some of the more serious patients from the festival.

On Saturday afternoon, the Rutherford Elementary School in Monticello was opened as a triage center to take pressure off the hospitals. Dr. Sydney Schiff, Chief of the Medical staff of CGH, was the medical coordinator for this emergency treatment center and made sure that enough physicians were on duty to treat patients at all times.

was sometimes chaotic, often improvised, but it was delivered in a professional and caring manner. Even the vaunted cases of recreational drug reactions were overblown and competently handled.

There were three explanations for this outcome. One was sheer good fortune. The second was the dedicated and selfless effort by both the paid staff and the countless volunteers who pitched in to help out over the course of the festival. The third was those very "vibes," the unique overflowing of good feelings that kept a crowd from turning into a mob.

Preparations

The promoters at Woodstock Ventures, sponsors of the festival, thought they had the perfect man to handle medical care. To begin with, Dr. William Abruzzi, 43, was local. He practiced general medicine in Wappingers Falls, NY, an hour-and-a-half east of the town of Bethel, where the concert would take place. He knew the lay of the land, was familiar with local hospitals.

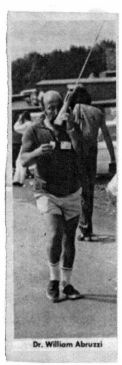

Dr. William Abruzzi

Abruzzi also had the needed experience. Having helped organize medical care at civil rights demonstrations in the South, he was something of an expert in "crowd medicine." He had cared for civil rights leader James Meredith and marched with Martin Luther King Jr.

Finally, he was simpatico. He understood the general philosophy that the promoters were pushing, which would later be referred to by the shorthand "peace and love."

As a bonus, Abruzzi had treated numerous drug cases while studying medicine at Columbia University in New York. He knew what he was doing and was not the type to call for the police or a straitjacket when confronted with a stoned teenager. Or to telephone the patient's parents.

Abruzzi himself felt the task would be straightforward. "I was asked to do something I've done several times before," he said.[7] His assignment was to set up health care facilities to handle 50,000 people for three days. From his experience, he figured two doctors, four nurses, and three assistants around the clock would do it.

Unfortunately, Abruzzi's preparations were based on an assumption known to be incorrect. Woodstock Ventures officials had hit on the number 50,000 when they approached the town fathers of Bethel even though they were virtually certain the festival would draw more. "I was planning on a quarter-million people," promoter Michael Lang said later, "but we didn't want to scare anyone."[8] Lang's disingenuousness would have consequences.

Woodstock Ventures promoters had hired Wesley Pomeroy as head of security. Given the widespread hostility felt toward the police by those expected to attend, the position was a delicate one. Pomeroy was the right man for the job, a 27-year veteran of law

The Age of Aquarius

The term Aquarius, the eleventh astrological sign of the zodiac, had been popularized by the rock musical Hair, which had arrived on Broadway in 1968 and was still playing during the Woodstock festival. The play's opening song declared *This is the dawning of the age of Aquarius.* Astrologers disputed when the 2,150-year era of Aquarius actually began, but hippies felt that something new must be getting underway, and in any case, it was a good excuse for a party. Woodstock promoters were inspired to call their event an "Aquarian Exposition."

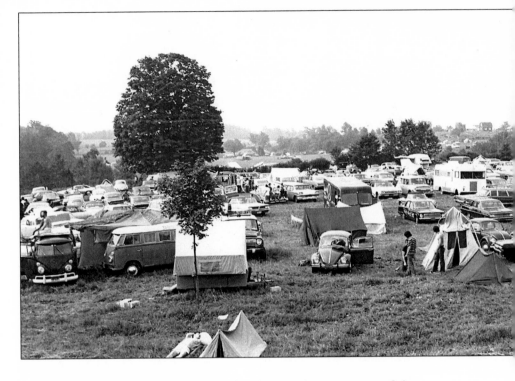

enforcement who had sympathy for the social movements of the day, a former Justice Department official, an ex-Marine who was friendly with radical comedian Dick Gregory.

Pomeroy was noted for his gentle and non-confrontational approach to crowd control and policing. He brought in Don Ganoung, an Episcopal priest who also had law enforcement experience, as his assistant. According to Pomeroy, Ganoung understood the "holistic dynamic of social interaction under stressful conditions."[9] On the official organization chart, Ganoung was the one responsible for the medical effort, with Dr. Abruzzi handling the actual operations.

Dr. Gustave Gavis, a Monticello pediatrician, was the acting Director of Health for the Town of Bethel. Three weeks in advance he went out to the site where the concert was scheduled to be held and saw what he thought were inadequate preparations. The promoters reassured him that things were under control. Again they

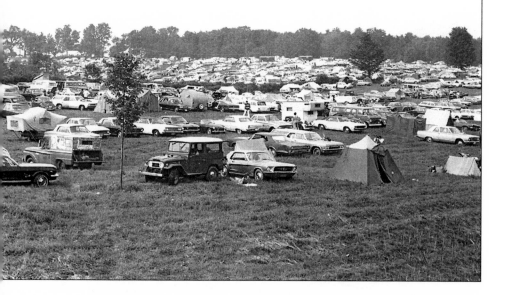

The first arrivals set up camp

mentioned numbers that appeared manageable. Gavis remembered later that "we expected around twenty to twenty-five thousand people, depending on the tickets that had been sold at that time."

Gavis was particularly concerned about the arrangements for water and sanitation, which he thought were inadequate. His experience with local secondary roads also gave him pause. "There were rocks on the road at that time.... I remember making house calls in that area, and it would kill your tires."[10]

Abruzzi arranged for 18 physicians, 36 nurses, 27 medical assistants in 8-hour shifts to cover the 72 hours of the festival. They would work in a trailer and a 30-bed hospital tent equipped with medications, first aid supplies, intravenous lines, and suturing kits. He ordered several gallons of Merthiolate, a trade name for thimerosal. This stinging, mercury-based topical antiseptic probably prevented many infections at the Woodstock Festival.

Mrs. Shirley Lowenthal's husband Stanley was the proprietor of Spector's Pharmacy, the largest in Monticello. She recalls representatives of Woodstock Ventures coming in several weeks before the festival to place large orders for various medications. "They ordered enough for Napoleon's army," she says.[11] The amount was so large that wholesalers required cash payments in advance.

Mrs. Lowenthal and her husband spent long nights filling hundreds of three-ounce bottles with cough syrup for festival-goers. She also sent in loads of Pampers disposable diapers and Enfamil baby formula, mostly for the young children of the members of the Hog Farm, the commune that was handling a variety of duties at the festival. All the supplies were airlifted from the parking lot of the Daitch Shopwell supermarket a few blocks from Spector's in

The State of Emergency Medical Services

The landmark National Highway Safety Act of 1966 introduced an overhaul of emergency medical services around the country. New systems of training and new standards for ambulances made important contributions to more efficient Emergency Medical Services (EMS). But the change did not happen overnight. In 1969, Emergency Medical Technicians (EMTs) did not yet routinely ride on ambulances – attendants were usually trained in Red Cross first aid, a less rigorous standard. Nor could ambulance personnel communicate directly with hospitals.

In some small towns, ambulance services were still provided by funeral home directors. The ambulances themselves were often based on Cadillac hearses and sported rakish fins. There was little room in back once a stretcher was on board, but those familiar with the vehicles attest to the comfortable ride. For the most part, these were the type of ambulance used at Woodstock.

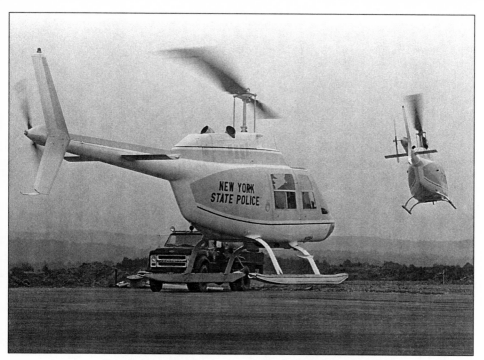

State Police using all means to maintain law, order, and health

Monticello, which served as a transfer point for some of the supplies being sent to the festival.

Abruzzi felt that with these medications and personnel, the situation was well in hand. The doctors would handle minor surgical procedures, and he made arrangements with Sullivan County Ambulance Service, a commercial company, to provide two regular ambulances and backups if needed. Medical people would communicate using twenty cumbersome walkie-talkie transceivers.

Doctors were to be paid $320 per shift, nurses $50, with an additional $17.50 to cover travel. A total of $15,875 was set aside to cover all medical costs for the festival.

The two divisions of Community General Hospital of Sullivan County in the nearby villages of Monticello and Liberty would handle more serious cases. Both hospitals called in extra people to work the weekend, doubling the usual staffing of their emergency

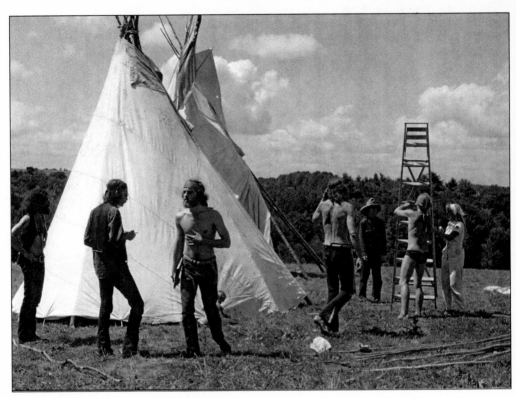

Hog Farmers setting up their medical tipis

rooms. Where possible, regular patients were discharged to free up beds. Uniformed deputy sheriffs or auxiliary police officers were stationed in each ER to keep order. In spite of Gavis's forebodings, preparations seemed adequate as the date of the festival approached.

Some had suggested manning the medical effort with volunteers, but Abruzzi felt that a paid staff was better. "Volunteers are great," he said, "but it becomes anarchistic."[12] He needed people under his command who would follow orders. He insisted the promoters provide the doctors with malpractice insurance.

"All of this seemed relatively routine," Abruzzi stated.[13] An official report later concurred that "Dr. Abruzzi planned well for 50,000 people."[14]

What's in a Name?

The term "Woodstock" has led to endless confusion about the 1969 festival to which it became indelibly attached. Woodstock is a town in Ulster County, New York. A well-known artist colony since at least the 1920s, it continues to attract musicians, artists, and eccentrics today. It's nestled in the eastern edge of the Catskill Mountains a little more than 100 miles due north of New York City.

The town wanted no part of the 1969 gathering and had no suitable venue for the 50,000 spectators it was expected to attract. But the name stuck. In part this was because of the cachet that went with "Woodstock," which at the time was the home of Bob Dylan, Jimi Hendrix, and other performers. The producers called themselves Woodstock Ventures and the event was the Woodstock Music and Art Fair even after its location shifted.

First nearby Saugerties, then the town of Wallkill, 30 miles closer to New York City, were considered. As the summer progressed, local opposition led to those plans falling through, and the promoters had to scramble to find yet another location. They settled on a remote tract of farm land in Bethel. That Sullivan County town sits in the southern foothills of the Catskills about 60 miles from the town of Woodstock. Bethel's best-known hamlet is White Lake; the closest substantial village is Monticello, ten miles from the festival site. Even before the festival had begun, hundreds of fair-goers showed up in the village of Woodstock, only to be redirected to the actual festival site.

Forty years later, the nomenclature is still creating confusion. Officials at the museum on the site of the original festival sponsored by the Bethel Woods Center for the Arts (http://www.bethelwoodscenter.org) regularly receive calls from visitors who are wandering around the village of Woodstock, looking for the museum dedicated to "Woodstock."

← SAUGERTIES 1
← WOODSTOCK 9
CAIRO 17 →

Dark Clouds

The problem was that the crowd slouching toward Bethel was, as Abruzzi put it, "frightening in its aspects."[15]

The oncoming masses caught Abruzzi by surprise. On Thursday one of the promoters had found the medical trailer padlocked even though it was supposed to be manned. Waiting outside were the weekend's first patients, a young couple who had been "ballin' all night."[16] The girl had forgotten her birth control pills and was hoping to pick up some.

The promoter called Abruzzi, who was still working at his own practice in Wappingers Falls. The doctor said his wife and a nurse named Betsey Morris were on their way, along with another nurse, Rikki Sanderson. Word was conveyed to the doctor that something like 85,000 spectators were in the process of arriving, with maybe 100,000 more on the way. Abruzzi said he would finish up and be right over.

Abruzzi understood that medical problems would not just double if the crowd doubled. More people could clog roads and prevent ambulance access. The crowding would multiply the likelihood of violence or panic. Overtaxed sanitation facilities could result in outbreaks of intestinal or other diseases. The number and severity of medical problems under such conditions could be much higher than predicted.

The good-natured, goateed doctor arrived at the site dressed in a Lacoste T-shirt and Bermuda shorts and quickly assessed the situation. He tripled his order of first aid supplies and tried to find additional ambulances. Thomas McFarlin, owner of Sullivan County Ambulance Service, had contracted to provide two ambulances on the grounds 24 hours a day for three days for a total of $600. He was asked to provide an additional ambulance on Thursday.

Until Abruzzi arrived, McFarlin's attendants performed first aid

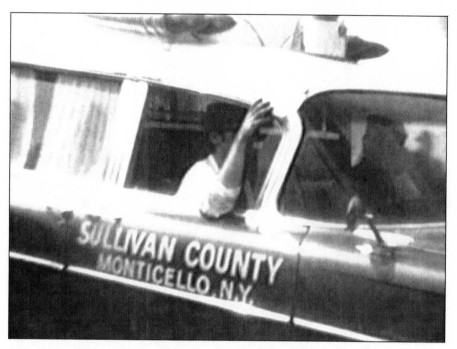

Ambulance crews on duty (a still from super 8 millimeter film)

on members of the already swelling crowd and took patients to local hospitals. When the roads became too clogged on Friday to take
patients out by road, the ambulances were used mainly on the site
itself to transport the injured to the hospital tent, or from there to
the helicopter pad.

Town of Liberty Volunteer Ambulance Corps (TOLVAC) personnel were on site with their ambulance for a while, but that left
Liberty with minimal coverage. Corps volunteer Carolyn Sprague
rode to the festival site with the ambulance, while members Paula
Bergman and Ida "Skippy" Frankel, among others, were brought
in via helicopter airlift from nearby Grossinger Airport, an effort
coordinated by Harold Lindsey of the Mamakating First Aid Squad
and Al Whittaker of the Woodbourne Fire Department First Aid
Squad. The men were officials of District 6 of the New York State
Volunteer Ambulance & First Aid Association, which served the
region.

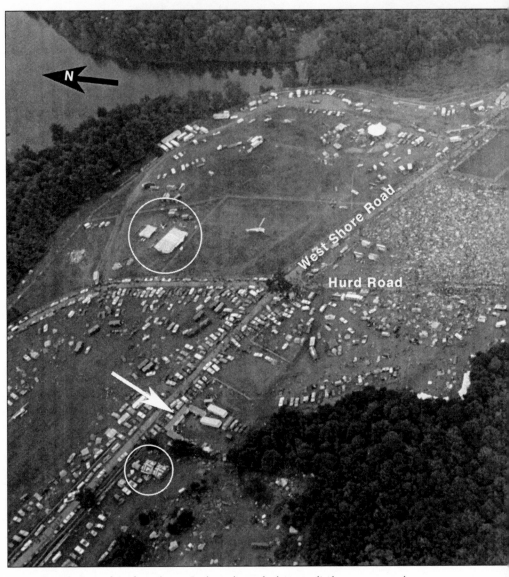

Aerial photo of the festival site. Circles indicate the large medical tent at top and small medical tents at bottom. Arrow shows the medical trailers in between. The main stage is out of view to the upper right.

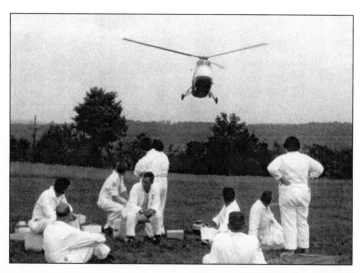

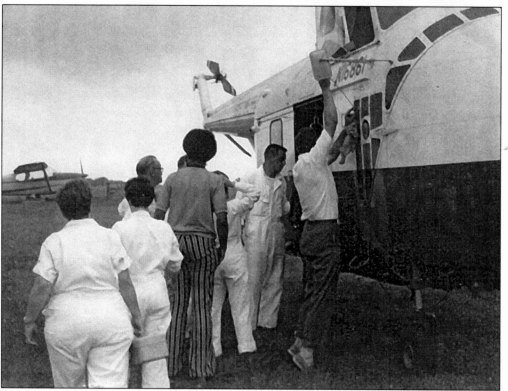

At Grossinger's Airport—ambulance volunteers and a drummer starting off to the festival

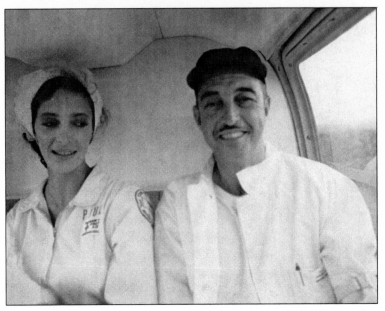

Paula Bergman, Town of Liberty Volunteer Ambulance Corp (TOLVAC), and Gerald Yager, Neversink Fire Department Volunteer Ambulance Corp on their way to the festival.

First aiders who volunteered with other local ambulance squads showed up to help, but left their ambulances home to provide for their communities. In addition to Al Whittaker, members of the Woodbourne Fire Department First Aid Squad who helped out included Charles Cohen, Sid Goldstein, and George Brown.

In many cases, the whole family pitched in. The husband and wife team of Gerald and Ruth Yager, members of the Neversink Fire Department First Aid Squad, flew in on Saturday afternoon and didn't leave till the next day. Ruth Baxter and her teenage son Michael, of the Mountaindale Fire Department First Aid Squad, came in by helicopter. George and Esther Boddy and their son Richard, from the Livingston Manor Volunteer Ambulance Corps, spent a day at the festival's medical tents. Jean Curry, also from Livingston Manor, flew in while her husband James, the Sullivan County Fire Coordinator, was establishing a countywide communications network for the mutual aid system and helping organize the county fire department response from the Control Center in Monticello.

In any case, the possibility of transporting patients by ambulance was diminishing. The only main road into the festival grounds was clogged for 15 miles. Moving critical patients out to hospitals would require helicopters.

As the crowd grew, the need for medical personnel increased as well. "We're understaffed," Abruzzi told a reporter. "Wait a minute, – did I say understaffed? I mean under siege."[17]

Word was put out for volunteers.

The hospitals themselves were already busy with the regular influx of vacationers. Sullivan County, where the festival was held, was a popular destination for visitors from the New York area. The horse racing track at Monticello and the numerous lakes and nearby mountains drew families to the area's resort hotels and bungalow colonies.

It seemed possible that medically the sky was falling, and there were many voices yelling that it was so. One was Dr. Donald Goldmacher, who had come to Woodstock as head of the Medical Committee on Human Rights New York Chapter. The volunteer group routinely provided doctors at civil rights and antiwar rallies and staffed a free clinic on New York City's lower East Side.

Dr. Goldmacher had made a deal with Woodstock Ventures executive Stanley Goldstein for the Committee to provide volunteer medical service at the festival in return for Woodstock Ventures donating to the group the medical equipment and supplies left over from the event.

But when he arrived on Saturday, the bearded New Yorker was aghast. "Nothing was there," he would remember. "It was a bad joke."[18]

Goldmacher was dismissive of Abruzzi's efforts. "He had no grasp of what was going on." It's more likely that Goldmacher was giving in to the anxiety that was overtaking many observers as they saw the potential for disaster looming larger with the growing crowds. "I was terrified," he admitted. "I was not prepared to see people die or needlessly get hurt or get sick."[19]

And still the Woodstock generation kept coming. Everyone knew that the situation now was out of control. John Roberts, one of the principal investors in Woodstock Ventures, noted, "There was nothing but the law of the – whatever the common will was, really. No one can enforce it."[20]

"How," Roberts asked, "do we control this beast that is out here?"

Earlier, Abruzzi had told Gordon Winarick, president of Monticello Hospital, "Don't worry. We've got it all under control."[21] But Winarick was afraid that if things went out of control, as they seemed ready to do, the burden would fall to local hospitals. He had consulted with authorities in Atlantic City, which earlier in the month had hosted a rock festival that grew a crowd of more than 100,000. He knew that a turnout three or four times as great could overwhelm facilities.

As the crowds grew, the idea of declaring the festival a disaster zone and using National Guard troops to clear the area was seriously considered. "They were stupid enough to believe they could mobilize the National Guard and move these kids out," said Woodstock Ventures production coordinator John Morris.[22]

And still they came.

"Why the hell aren't they stopping them?" asked the worried Dr. Goldmacher. "I don't want to verbalize how bad this thing could be if they kept coming. They have got to be stopped."[23]

Hog Farm

One area of relative calm in this increasingly nervous situation was the New Mexico commune called the Hog Farm and its leader, counterculture stalwart Hugh Romney, who would go down in history as Wavy Gravy, a name he acquired later. Eighty-five Hog Farmers, pranksters in the best hippie tradition, had been hired by Woodstock Ventures and flown to New York two weeks early.

"We brought in the Hog Farm to be our crowd interface," said Woodstock Ventures operative Stanley Goldstein. "We needed a specific group to be the exemplars for all to follow. We believed that the idea of sleeping outdoors under the stars would be very attractive to many people, but we knew damn well that the kind of people who were coming had never slept under the stars in their lives. We had to create a circumstance where they were cared for."[24]

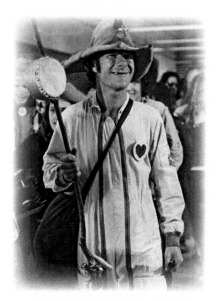

Wavy Gravy in action

Their duties would include building and shopping for a free food kitchen, setting up the nature trails, and helping city kids learn the basics of camping. They were to take care of lost babies, help campers build fires at the campgrounds. Afterward, they would be on the clean-up detail. They would also have a role in security – they would be the event's "please force."

"My God, we're the cops! I can't believe it!" Wavy Gravy marveled. On learning the group's duties were to include security, he said he planned to used lemon pies and seltzer bottles for crowd control.[25] Security actually meant establishing a mood for the festival, and it was a job the Hog Farmers performed superbly.

"These people were asked to come because they can serve the needs of the crowd and solve any problems in communication," a festival spokesman pointed out. "If someone gets sick, they will be there to help if someone can't relate to a doctor in a white uniform."[26] Hog Farm members were identified by red arm bands with a stamp depicting a winged pig – more of these bands were created for the volunteers from the audience who joined the Hog Farm effort. "The farmers were sweeping people out of the fields," Wavy Gravy said, "and we would incorporate them into our work crews."[27]

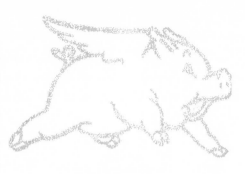

Their responsibilities in the medical realm proved to be the group's main contribution to the Woodstock Festival. In particular, they helped manage the hundreds of bad trips and freakouts that the weekend became famous for.

The Hog Farmers had accumulated plenty of first-hand experience with psychedelic drugs. What's more, Hog Farm members Lisa and Tom Law and others had run a "trip tent" at the Monterey Pop festival two years before. There they had developed a technique of helping those whose acid trips had taken a turn down queer street.

Many credit the Hog Farm with saving Woodstock. From a medical perspective, their experience and good judgement in dealing with hundreds of patients experiencing bad trips removed a burden from overworked doctors and nurses. And their approach was beneficial for patients who would otherwise have required sedation.

Volunteers Step Up

On Friday, the situation at the festival grounds was becoming dire. Only two doctors had managed to arrive – many were stuck in traffic. Supplies were running low.

Around this time, the real spirit of Woodstock began to infuse the medical effort. Abruzzi had worried about anarchy if volunteers provided the bulk of the service, but now he had no choice.

Dr. Desmond Callan, one of the founders of the Medical Committee for Human Rights, did not travel to Woodstock with that group but instead was headed toward a weekend vacation in upstate New York. On his way, he heard a radio report that physicians were desperately needed. Anxious to help, he turned around and drove to Bethel. On arrival he found that the situation was not the crisis that had been described, but he decided to stay and help out.

Another who answered the call for doctors was Dr. Albert P. Sutton of Great Neck, who had been visiting friends in Middletown, 35 miles from Bethel. His son Ira was attending the festival. "They need all the help they can get," he decided.[28]

Sutton was flown into the site on a mid-sized five-place helicopter along with other physicians and some additional supplies. With him was Dr. Anibal Herrera, a psychiatrist who picked up a supply of the tranquilizers Thorazine, Mellaril, and Valium from the psychiatric hospital in Middletown, where he was on staff.

Sutton later remembered:

> On arrival we were taken to a trailer used by Dr. Abruzzi, then I was taken to a tent used as an emergency room which was run by a group of people called Hog Farmers, along with Abbie Hoffman, who I then met. There were adequate supplies; plenty of food trucked in from New York City, but a shortage of ice for medications, which were brought in by helicopter. ... I remember girls complaining of cystitis, crazy sex activities.... LSD was present and it was claimed that it was dumped into drinks, some people were sent on TRIPS and they went crazy and wild. The psychiatrists would not use Thorazine but Abbie Hoffman's group were able to talk them down until they became lucid.[29]

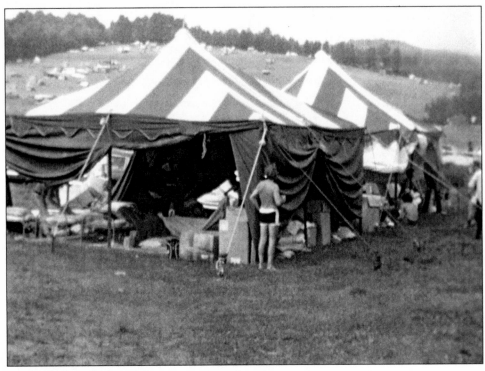

Small medical tent, well-stocked, waiting for the rush

The tent that Sutton refers to was a large circus tent that had originally been intended as the mess tent for festival employees. Located near the helicopter landing zone, it was commandeered to become the main field hospital in order to absorb the overflow from Dr. Abruzzi's first-aid trailers and smaller tent. Both facilities were supplemented by 11 first aid stations manned by nurses scattered around the festival grounds.

Because of its pink and white stripes, most of the medical people took to calling the tent "Big Pink" or the "Pink and White." On Friday evening, just before Joan Baez appeared on the main stage, volunteers and medical workers cleared out the tables and installed about 100 cots. The tent divided into a freakout area and a medical area, with a small section reserved where medical people could try to catch some sleep. During at least part of the festival, a deputy sheriff was assigned there to guard medical supplies.

Much of the help emerged from the crowd itself. Dr. Peter Uhlmann had come to the festival to enjoy the concert with his wife and her sisters. Just after the music began on Friday, he noticed a young man behind him in the crowd having an apparent seizure.

"He was probably in his teens and was not responding to verbal cues," Uhlmann wrote later. "I was told a medical tent existed nearby and several of us carried him there."

A doctor in the tent, burdened by the increasing flow of patients, asked Uhlmann to stay and help.

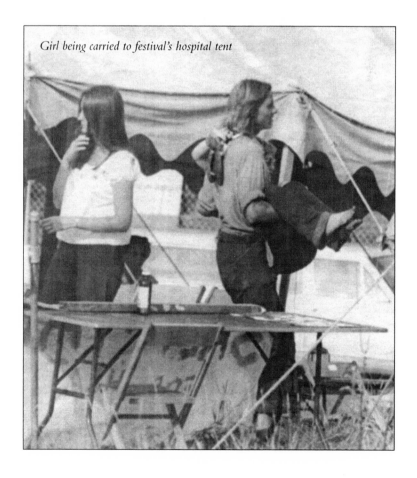

Girl being carried to festival's hospital tent

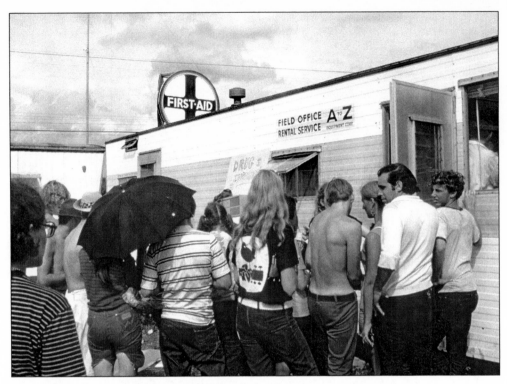

The walking wounded lined up at the medical trailer...

"After examining the young man we had carried in," he reported, "it was decided his symptoms were the result of a bad trip. His most bizarre behavior was pursing his lips and blowing against them. This activity was so extreme he actually caused the soft tissues of his neck to swell from subcutaneous emphysema. None of us had seen this before and were concerned he might actually require a tracheostomy, which we were not prepared to perform under those circumstances. Fortunately, it was not necessary and he slowly improved as the drugs were eliminated from his system."

A young woman came into the tent with an acute abdomen, severe pain that alerted doctors to the possibility of appendicitis, ulcer or ectopic pregnancy. Again the diagnosis was a negative reaction to drugs. Only supportive care was needed.

"In my brief experience as a doctor I had not seen so many

drug reactions that mimicked physical illness," Uhlmann noted. He had completed an internship at a busy urban hospital in Oakland, California, and had seen his share of drug cases. But patients there usually presented with psychological symptoms, ranging from hallucinations to paranoia, rather than physical complaints.

Uhlmann himself had experimented with marijuana and psychedelic drugs, and he was asked to take charge of patients coming in with drug-related issues. "In most cases, I made a diagnosis, provided reassurance and then forwarded the patients to the 'trip tent.'"

The doctor was impressed with the talk-down treatment offered by Hog Farm members, who were able to keep trippers' minds occupied with positive thoughts. "I don't recall having to sedate patients with benzodiazepines [Valium] or phenothiazines

...and some could walk no more.

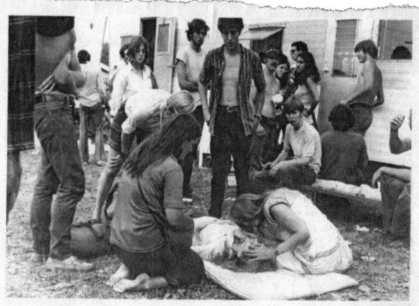

An unidentified girl, one of hundreds of the youngsters at the Aquarian Festival who have "freaked-out," is given some loving care at the site's first aid station. A freak-out, in hip lingo, is a violent physical and mental withdrawal reaction from drugs or other stimulus.

[Thorazine], which was the recommended medical approach at the time. Also, there was a danger in mixing sedatives with unknown chemicals. We didn't want to cause more problems by creating drug interactions."[30]

Uhlmann spent the entire festival in the medical tent, saw no bands, and spent little time with his family. Half a year later he received a check from one of the doctors he had worked with, he said in a 2009 interview. The $50 was to reimburse him for the price of his ticket.

"I was a first-year medical student spending my vacation in the area," remembered surgeon Kenneth Steinglass. "I ended up staying and acting as a doctor, using a walkie-talkie to talk to real doctors for advice. I'll never forget walking back to my car at one a.m. Friday night. It was very still and had just stopped raining. Joan Baez was singing 'Swing Low, Sweet Chariot' almost half a mile away, and her voice carried across Fillipini Pond. The purity of her voice and the stillness of the night remain with me to this day."[31]

Meanwhile, political activist Abbie Hoffman was growing increasingly worried. Hoffman, then 32, had long been a leader of civil rights and anti-war efforts. He was a founder of the Youth International Party, or Yippies, who specialized in political theater, such as throwing dollar bills onto the floor of the New York Stock Exchange or attempting to "levitate" the Pentagon during a 1967 demonstration. At the time of the festival he was under indictment for his part in the disturbances at the Chicago Democratic convention the year before.

He had expressed concerns during the summer that the promoters were planning a "capitalist rip-off" of festival-goers and threatened to disrupt the event with the help of his radical cohorts from New York's Lower East Side. The promoters decided it was prudent to include Hoffman in the process and to pay him to put out a "survival sheet" that would help festival participants to find services. Security chief Pomeroy listened to Hoffman's advice on needed medical supplies and assigned him and his people some radios. "We were defusing them, that's all," Pomeroy stated later.[32]

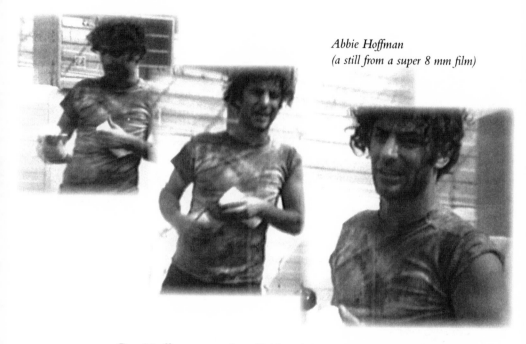

Abbie Hoffman
(a still from a super 8 mm film)

But Hoffman sensed on Friday there was serious trouble brewing. He pressed the promoters for more doctors, more supplies. "It was one of my best organizing moments," he remembered about bringing some order to the medical volunteers.[33]

Hoffman's "ol man" had run a medical supply business, where the activist had worked as a teenager. Abbie himself had a master's degree in psychology. He had taken a job as a psychologist in a state psychiatric hospital and put in a stint as a pharmaceutical salesman. This background, leavened by abundant self-confidence, inspired Hoffman to take a hand and help administer the medical effort.

Possessed of a dynamic personality, Hoffman went into a whirlwind of organizing. He assigned roles to the volunteers who were flooding in, helped convert the pink mess tent for medical care.

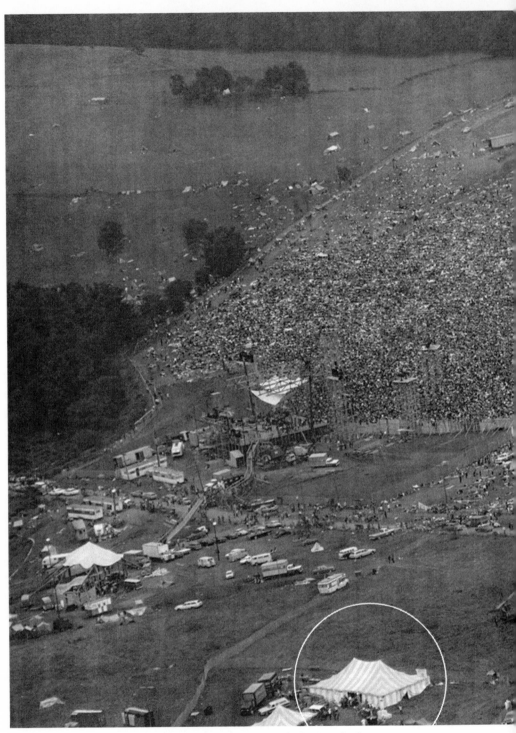

Circles indicate the large "pink and white" medical tent...

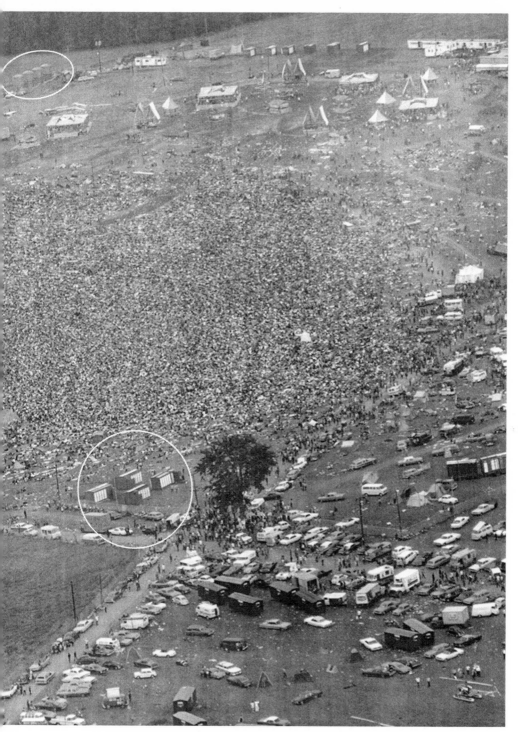

...and some of the portable toilets. Ellipse at top highlights water tanks

Plain army cots without sheets or mattresses were available. Some patients had to settle for plastic sheets on the grass. Hoffman posted signs directing patients to "Waiting Room," "Admissions," "Volunteers," or "Rest Area."

The organizer instilled drama and politics into everything. He didn't just go off to collect medical supplies from the trailers for the tent; he was "stealing" them. He wasn't just helping out; he said, "I'm just trying to prevent disaster from occurring. I'm trying to save lives."[34]

Hoffman worked with a "really cool-headed gal named Jill who had been an Army supply nurse," to order additional supplies.[35] He also encountered George, a local resident who coordinated ambulances. He gave the personnel fanciful names like "William Head Doctor," "Sid Cuts," "Lee Heat Tablets." Liberty Ambulance volunteer Skippy Frankel was appointed Registrar of his newly founded hospital.

He thought his father would appreciate the irony. "I was finally settling in the Hospital Business."[36]

Chaos

On Saturday, Dr. Sydney P. Schiff, a surgeon from Liberty who was the Chief of Staff at Community General Hospital and also Chief Medical Officer for Civil Defense in Sullivan County was asked to survey the situation. Confused reports were coming in as reporters phoned local officials to try to chase down rumors. Schiff's report reflects some of the sense of chaos and disorder that reigned.

"There were frantic requests being made for food, water, medical supplies," Schiff recounted. "There was no real order or discipline in the area. I had the feeling almost of a great natural disaster affecting a large city with no organizing or control. . . . Throughout this episode, in our dealings with the people at the festival, the panic button was constantly being pushed....Everybody seemed to want to jump into a helicopter and ride around and issue orders and make requests."[37]

He observed a hot, crowded medical trailer without proper instruments or proper set-up. Long lines of young people waited patiently for treatment.

Schiff never got to the pink tent where many of the drug cases were being treated, but said, "I would hear conflicting reports. Reports of 'dedicated people' and reports of incredible filth and primitive conditions with complete lack of organization or anything resembling a proper type of medical field facility."[38]

Dr. Abruzzi, Schiff reported, was constantly calling to requisition supplies throughout the county. The local hospitals were already overburdened. "This was the middle of August, and we were at the height of our busy season," Schiff noted. "Our medical and hospital staffs were already exhausted with their own work and the season, let alone THIS disaster."[39]

A newspaper reporter sent his editor the message that, "Ambulance from the site to Monticello Community Hospital, normally a 15-minute run, took more than two hours to bring a patient in with an injured leg. Hospital officials worried to say the least."[40]

At that point, everyone involved in the medical effort at Woodstock was worried. To say the least.

"Announcement From the Stage

This is one thing I was gonna wait a while before we talked about, maybe we can talk about it. It's a free concert from now on. That doesn't mean anything goes. We're gonna put the music up here for free. Now let's face the situation. We've had thousands and thousands of people show up here today, many more than we knew or thought would be possible. We're gonna need each other to help each other to work this out, 'cause of systems we worked out. We're gonna bring the food in. The one major thing you've go to remember at night when you go back up to the woods to go to sleep or you stay here, is that the man next to you is your brother and you damn well better treat each other that way. Because if you don't, we blow the whole thing. But we've got it right there. "

2

Into the Maelstrom

While the metaphorical storm was gathering around the festival, real storms hit the area with a vengeance. Friday night saw heavy showers. Saturday morning, a downpour turned the worn pasture land and newly bulldozed roads into a sea of mud. Mud became the "fifth element" of the festival.

The conditions escalated the potential for a medical disaster. The mud sucked sneakers and sandals from the feet of many who weren't already barefoot and at the same time hid broken glass, loose pop tops, and other debris. An epidemic of cut feet was unavoidable. "Almost every other case which appeared for first aid was a case of foot injury or foot laceration and/or puncture wound," Dr. Abruzzi reported afterward.[1]

And since this was a working farm with a usual complement of manure, the risk of infection was grave. Doctors were particularly concerned about tetanus – a potentially fatal illness.

In spite of daytime temperatures in the 90s, drenched clothing raised the risk of hypothermia especially at night. The conditions

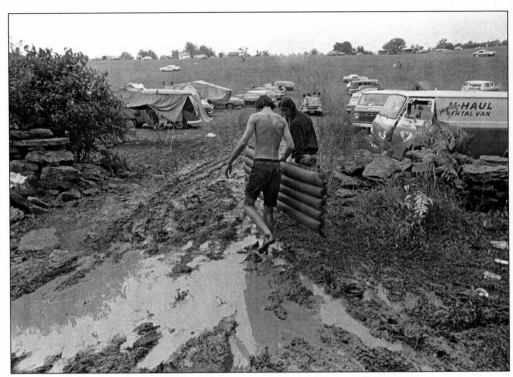

Mud, the "fifth element" of the festival   *Opposite: Bad scene, good care*

significantly increased the psychological strain on the crowd. Living in soggy, dirty surroundings prompted fair-goers to approach townspeople and beg for a chance to shower. The dense crowds themselves gave some spectators fits of anxiety and claustrophobia.

Bad drug reactions began to pile up. A contemporary newspaper account said Abruzzi handled "25 freakouts an hour from LSD-type drugs Friday night."[2] His staff, it was reported, had handled at least 1,000 patients from all causes during the first 24 hours of the festival.

And still they came. By early afternoon on Saturday, the New York State Police were estimating a crowd of 400,000 was already at the festival grounds. Others said an additional half million young people were on the road heading for the place that had suddenly become "the place to be." Bus lines at New York's Port Authority stopped selling tickets to any of the surrounding towns. "We're not driving into that disaster area," said a spokesman for Short Line Bus Company.[3]

Troopers closed the New York Thruway exits with the most convenient access to the festival. Drivers who were on their way to Woodstock were told to turn back as far away as the Canadian border, 300 miles distant. The Toronto *Globe & Mail* reported that two buses carrying 107 Canadians were stopped by immigration authorities in Buffalo, N.Y., who claimed the passengers were under the influence of drugs.[4]

The medical situation at the festival now hung in the balance. By late Friday, hospitals in Liberty and Monticello were full. The larger Horton Hospital in Middletown was admitting some of the more serious cases. Liz Hermann, then a staff nurse at the thirty-bed Ellenville Hospital in Ulster County, 30 miles from the site, remembers even her facility being put on alert, though they received no patients.

A radio announcement was broadcast by Dr. Donald Goldmacher

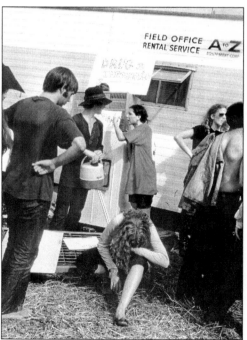

requesting "hip doctors" and supplies of tranquilizers and anti-spasmodics. Newspapers were reporting patients "writhing on ground from overdoses." The smell in the air was "Egyptian filth," commented local congressman Martin B. McKneally, who flew over the site (McKneally, who was in high dudgeon over the festival, asserted that "the stench that arose from the hill on Yasgur farm will remain in the nostrils of the people of Sullivan County for years to come.")[5]

Two Are Dead...

Two are dead and two are supposedly in critical condition, one from an attempt to set himself on fire and one from an overdose of drugs. Confirmation on this is difficult due to lack of communication between the site and officials. The latest on traffic is that the area is still congested and that traffic is not moving into the area. The only traffic that is moving is away from the area.

—*George Spicka on WELV radio (Ellenville, New York) for the Mutual Broadcasting System Network*

Some of the reports were exaggerated, but the danger was real. One of the volunteers at a tent that provided counseling and legal aid noted that many in the crowd were "people who don't know what to do when they decide to spend three days living in the woods."[6]

By Saturday night the medical tents were treating an average of 200 patients every hour. A long line stretched outside Dr. Abruzzi's first aid trailer. Some helicopter pilots had already been going for twenty hours without a rest. Tetanus toxoid ran low and emergency calls went out for the crucial vaccine. "Almost every available vial of tetanus toxoid in Sullivan County was utilized for our purposes," Abruzzi reported afterward.[7]

Care was given in less than ideal conditions. Movement of patients to the medical facilities was hampered by the dense crowds, rough terrain, and mud. A U-Haul pickup truck equipped with two cots in the back and driven by a teenager with shaky skills on a stick shift was used as an ambulance. He lurched around the grounds while his assistants made siren sounds.

One of those assistants reported picking up a woman who was breathing but "appeared to be unconscious or something. She wasn't awake." Back at the hospital tent she woke up and "said she passed out because she had to go to the bathroom so bad." Another patient had a "this thing on the side of his cheek the size of a baseball – an abscess, I think." He had taken more than a dozen pills since Friday and was "definitely having some problems."[8]

Volunteers

In response to Goldmacher's urgent plea and other appeals broadcast over radio stations in New York City, volunteer doctors headed toward Bethel to help out at the festival. One who responded was Dr. Sam V. Boor, an ear-nose-and-throat specialist in private practice in the city. Following the broadcast instructions, he drove to New York's LaGuardia Airport and, with a couple of other doctors, was whisked to Bethel in a helicopter.

Hog Farmers preparing food for the crowd — vegetarian, of course

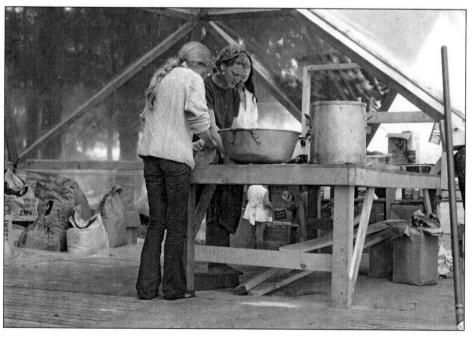

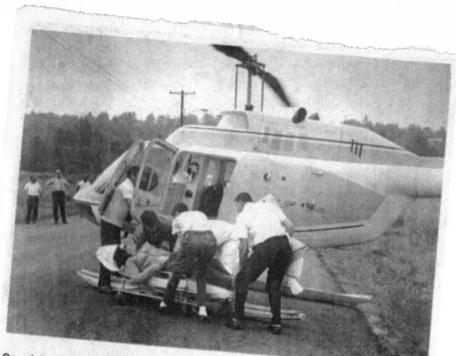

One of the weekend's many striken youths at the Aquarian Festival is helped into a helicopter by emergency attendants on roadway near the White Lake festival site.

TH-Record photo

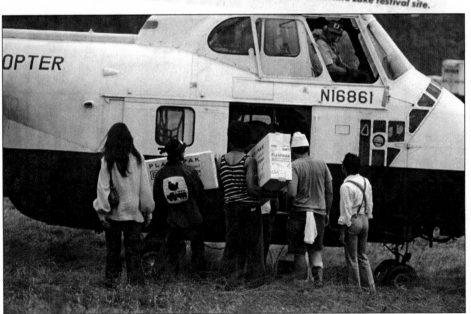

Helicopters became essential to get supplies in and people out of the festival.

On arrival he was "taken to a huge tent with hundreds of young people milling around, a scene of confusion." He would spend the next two days there.

"I'll never forget that scene," he remembered later, "literally hundreds of screaming kids carried to our tent, sedated with Valium and transported by military helicopter (out to the Rutherford School)."

Boor was impressed by the techniques and leadership role of Wavy Gravy and felt that the presence of the Hog Farm "saved the day." He followed instructions from an Australian psychiatrist who had used LSD in his practice. This doctor, Boor said, explained how to treat bad trips with intravenous Valium rather than Thorazine.

Presented with a screaming tripper, "first the farmers would try the talking cure and if that didn't work, send them to the tent where we started IVs if no other problem appeared present and give small doses of IV Valium per our psychiatrist's protocol. Other Hog Farmers would hold the patient's hand and the patient fell into a deep sleep."

Announcement From the Stage

Alan Fay, go to the information booth, your friend is very sick. Alan Fay, please go to the information booth, man.

Then Air Force medics would pick up the sedated patients and transport them by helicopter to the Rutherford School where they would sleep off the Valium. Boor accompanied one of the flights to assure himself of the outcome of this treatment by examining patients at the school.

"It all came together by hook and crook with the help of volunteers, the Hog Farm and the military," Boor acknowledged.[9]

Others who pitched in to help were citizens' band radio operators. CB radios were used by truck drivers, plumbers, delivery people, and a few hobbyists for short-range mobile communications (they would become wildly popular in the 1970s).

Liberty News columnist Jeff Blumenfeld reported later that thanks to the dedication of 37 citizens' band operators and five ham radio buffs, "additional food and volunteers were sent to de Hoyos Park and to the Rutherford School Hospital." Traffic reports circulated on these airwaves as well, and "ambulances were dispatched sooner than would have been possible without calls from mobile units at the scenes."[10]

A CB enthusiast named Tom (KBY 5014) was caught in traffic on Route 17. He kept his car running and stayed on the air almost continuously for two days, relaying information from the Sullivan County Civil Defense office in Monticello about traffic and the soup kitchen in town. Blumenfeld himself helped man this communications center after assigned Civil Defense officials abandoned their efforts.[11]

Death

Given the crowds and conditions, it was expected that fatalities would be unavoidable at the Woodstock Festival. Some pointed out that the gathering had grown to the proportions of Buffalo, which at 462,000 inhabitants was the second largest city in New York State.

In a population that size, more than two dozen deaths would be typical over a three-day period. In fact, 40 deaths were recorded in Buffalo that weekend (Rochester, the state's next largest city, saw 33 die out of a population of 296,000).

On the one hand, Woodstock attendees were overwhelmingly young and healthy. But accidents normally account for 5% of all deaths, and the potential for motor vehicle crashes, drownings, electrocutions, fall, and violence was high at the festival. The weather – rain, lightning, high wind gusts – was a further peril, and widespread drug use added another dangerous element to the mix.

The fact that the expected rash of deaths did not materialize was a blessing; the fact that two teenagers did die was a deep tragedy.

The first fatality came at 10:30 a.m. Saturday morning. Raymond R. Mizsak, a seventeen-year-old from Trenton, N.J., was asleep in a sleeping bag beside Hurd Road on the festival grounds. A tractor pulling a wagon with a tank for pumping out the portable latrines ran over Mizsak's chest. Ambulance attendants picked him up and took him to a first aid station. Doctors called for a helicopter.

"Doctors pumped air into him with a small hand pump," a reporter stated. "His face was puffed and bluish; blood trickled from the corner of his mouth."[12]

By the time a helicopter landed twenty minutes later, a blood-soaked towel covered Mizsak's head. He was dead. The helicopter took an injured girl instead. An ambulance removed the body of the dead boy.

"It was a real heavy trip," noted Tom Law, the Hog Farmer who had held the boy in his arms.[13]

Carol Green, a cook for Woodstock Ventures, expressed the feeling of many: "I never thought that there would be any death... I was just bereft that someone should die there."[14]

Saturday night brought the second death of the festival. Richard Beiler, an eighteen-year-old Marine from Long Island was slated to leave soon for Vietnam. He decided to take in the festival while at home on leave and headed up to Bethel with friends. His cousin Bryan St. Louis observed later that Beiler "may have been the only short-haired guy there."[15]

Beiler became ill Saturday night. He was carried into the hospital tent unconscious. Doctors ordered him to be airlifted to the triage center in Monticello by helicopter.

Deputy Phillip Key, who was Sullivan County Sheriff Louis R. Ratner's driver, reported, "As a chopper approached the landing area I saw Sheriff Ratner and a doctor desperately administering artificial respiration to a young boy. Upon landing he was rushed into an ambulance, his two legs held high trying to keep him alive. I was later told that all efforts were to no avail."[16] Elevation of the legs was a standard treatment for a patient experiencing signs of shock.

From the Rutherford School, Beiler was transported by Sullivan County Ambulance Service 25 miles to Middletown's Horton Memorial Hospital, which lacked a helicopter landing pad. He arrived at Horton still unconscious at 11:00 p.m. He was declared dead at 6:35 a.m. Sunday morning. Orange County Coroner Kenneth March, who directed the autopsy, suspected Beiler had died of an overdose of drugs, probably heroin. A definitive cause of death had to await toxicology tests.

Because of March's initial suspicion, most subsequent accounts of the Woodstock Festival attributed Beiler's death to heroin use. But one of those who treated Beiler was the volunteer doctor, Sam Boor. His account of the incident raises questions about the actual cause of death:

> Boor remembered "a kid who was brought to the hog farmers screaming and just 'out of it.' Hugh [Romney] correctly knew the patient was sicker than just a 'bad trip' and brought him directly to the medical tent where I assumed his care. The first thing we noted, other than being really semi-comatose, was that he had a temperature over 104 degrees Fahrenheit. We started an IV and transported him to the school with me in attendance. From there we took him via ambulance to the nearest big hospital in [Middletown] where the attending MD took charge. On the way, he had arrest of breathing and was intubated and bagged. I returned to the festival grounds but a few days later called the hospital and found that he had died, the autopsy showed myocarditis. Putting the history and physical findings together makes me wonder if he actually

had hyperthermia and could have been saved. I wasn't familiar with that syndrome at the time, but someone taking LSD and then getting Thorazine can develop hyperthermia and go on to die unless steps are taken to lower his body temp which wasn't done to my knowledge."[17]

Hyperthermia, the medical term for a dangerously elevated body temperature, can be a side effect that sometimes accompanies the administration of Thorazine. Both LSD and methamphetamine can also cause high fever.

Myocarditis, a sometimes fatal inflamation of the heart muscle, can be caused by fever, or by infection or toxic chemicals. Boor's account is suggestive that something other than a simple heroin overdose might have been responsible for Beiler's death. With autopsy records sealed, a definitive explanation remains elusive.

Injury

A number of festival participants were seriously injured. One man was found unconscious in the wee hours of Sunday morning and brought to Dr. Abruzzi, who recognized that the man was in serious

---

Diagnoses

Patients from the festival who were admitted to Liberty branch of Community General Hospital:

Pelvic Inflammatory Disease	Several lacerations of forehead, possible concussion
Possible fractured skull	Possible meningitis
Multiple body injuries	Hysterical reaction
Overdose of drugs, possible concussion	Possible fractured skull, cerebral concussion
Massive laceration left side of forehead	
Contusions of right shoulder	

Fractured left clavicle

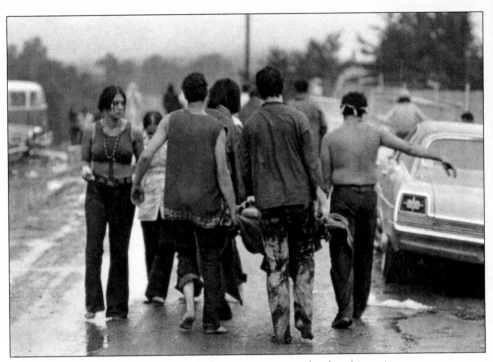

Volunteers lend a hand.   *Opposite: Tempting fate for a better view*

condition. He ordered the patient to be flown immediately to Horton Hospital, the closest facility with an intensive care unit. The patient, he was sure, hovered close to death.

Two other patients were awaiting airlift, one with a possible case of appendicitis, the other with a broken ankle. But Abruzzi insisted that his serious case go out first.

Around 2:30 a.m. a helicopter landed but the pilot reported that he only had enough fuel to fly to the facility at Monticello. No one was around to pump fuel at the airport.

Abruzzi insisted that "the man is near death . . . and in fourth degree cardiac failure," and needed the artificial kidney machine that was available at Horton. "I don't think we can wait more than 15 minutes," Abruzzi said. "He just won't make it."[18]

Another helicopter was ordered from Grossinger's Resort in Liberty, New York, ten miles away. The Catskill hotel had a small airport and was the transfer point for the musicians being flown into the festival. This helicopter set down in the landing zone marked by red Christmas tree bulbs. But a communications error resulted in the man being flown to Monticello aboard the first chopper.

Though the second helicopter was sent to transport him from Monticello, there was apparently confusion about whether Horton could receive airlifted patients – it could not. In any case, the patient arrived there by ambulance at 5:30 a.m. Diagnosed with acute alcohol poisoning, his stomach was pumped and he was put on dialysis. He recovered and was able to be sent home two days later.

Other serious injuries occurred. George Xikis, 18, of New York City fractured his skull when he fell from the car roof while under influence of drugs, it was reported.[19]

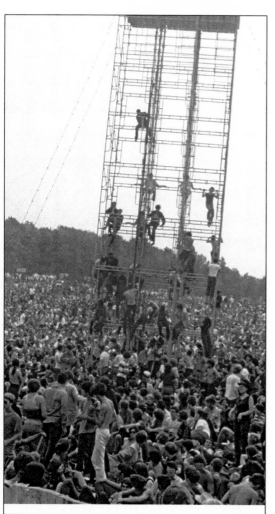

One fair-goer was trying to build a fire using a can of lighter fluid with a hole in the bottom. The fluid dripped on his foot and caught fire. Struggling to put out the flames he got more fluid on himself. He received burns to the upper part of his body and face. He wound up in intensive care in St. Luke's Hospital, Newburgh, N.Y.

A newspaper reported that "one youth, reportedly under the influence of drugs, climbed a sound tower near center stage and plunged 60 feet to the ground, breaking his back." He had to be evacuated by helicopter.[20]

Sheriff's Deputy Michael Rothman reported: "An injured girl was on the side of the road. She had fallen off a car, sustaining damage to her right temple, and abrasions on various parts of her body. She was lifted into the ambulance and Dep. Rothman then showed the ambulance driver the way to Route 55 and on to the hospital in Liberty."

Dr. Sydney Schiff remembered seeing "cases where young people had fallen from moving vehicles onto their heads, necks, arms, and legs, with injuries to these areas. I saw one boy that had been crushed between two trucks, who incredibly did not suffer anything but multiple lacerations of his trunk."[21]

Dr. Goldmacher ordered a woman suffering from hepatitis to be airlifted to Schenectady General Hospital, almost 130 miles away, at 6:00 p.m. Sunday.

One young woman being delivered by helicopter to the hospital in Monticello kept screaming in pain from what might have been appendicitis. When the nurse taking over her care asked her, "Where does it hurt?" she said, "'Where do you think it hurts? I have the clap.'"[22]

A deputy reported, "I picked up Dr. Abruzzi at West Shore and Hurd and transported him to Perry and West Shore where he stitched up the head of a boy who had fallen off the roof of a car. The boy was then transported to the hospital tent by a truck which I escorted."[23]

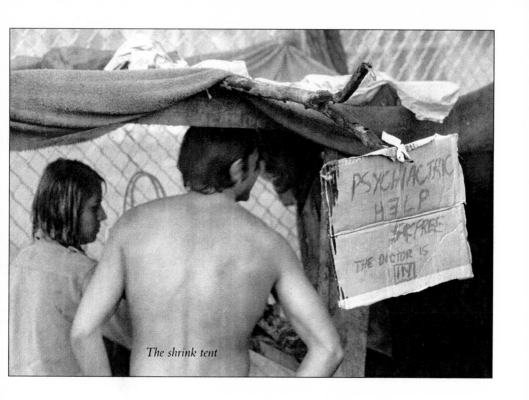

The shrink tent

The Big Freakout

No medical situation at Woodstock drew as much attention or presented as unique a set of problems as did the use of recreational drugs. The drug subculture was well established in America at the time of the festival, and the battalions who arrived at Bethel were its foot soldiers. Several of the groups on the bill – including Jefferson Airplane, the Grateful Dead, and Jimi Hendrix – were originators of what was called "acid rock," music that celebrated chemical mind alteration and included long improvised instrumental solos.

"Most of the rock music nowadays is played by stoned people for stoned people," said one concert-goer.[24]

Drugs weren't just available, a regular drug bazaar was operating in one wooded area of the grounds throughout the festival. Prices were posted on trees. Marijuana, which was in short supply

Chemical Recreation

Marijuana   Many observers reported that the air at Woodstock was heavily scented with the smell of burning *Cannabis sativa*. Its medical significance was minimal except for a few volunteer nurses who reported feeling "high," just from breathing the air.

LSD   Lysergic acid diethylamide was the most popular psychedelic in use at the festival. Synthesized from the grain fungus ergot in 1938, LSD burst into the headlines in 1967. By the time of the Woodstock festival the drug had attracted a mass following of casual users. Among its physical effects were dilated pupils, jaw clenching, and sometimes fever, weakness or nausea. Its main dangers were psychological, including sensual distortion, hallucination, and emotional reactions.

Mescaline   A natural psychedelic derived from the peyote cactus and used by Native Americans for centuries. Its effects were similar to LSD, with intense visual hallucinations. The effects lasted from 6 to 12 hours.

Psilocybin   An extract of mushrooms of the *Psilocybe* genus. Another potent hallucinogen, its effects were described by some users as more "spiritual" than drugs like LSD.

MDA   There were some reports of methylenedioxyamphetamine use at Woodstock. The drug (a relative of "Ecstacy") was a psychedelic, but unlike LSD it was toxic in large doses. Symptoms of acute toxicity could include agitation, sweating, increased blood pressure and heart rate, dramatic increase in body temperature, and convulsions. Overdoses could be fatal.

Heroin   A morphine derivative, heroin produced euphoria and relaxation. It had the potential to slow the heartbeat and breathing and drop blood pressure, resulting in death. Heroin was particularly dangerous when combined with alcohol. Naloxone, now the standard antidote for opiate overdose was not yet available at the time of the Woodstock Festival.

Speed   Methamphetamine, also known as Methedrine, is a powerful central nervous system stimulant and was used recreationally for the euphoria and energy that it gave users. Physically it raised blood pressure and heart rate. Excessive talking was a common symptom. The danger of heart attack or stroke had led to the mantra "speed kills." It was sometimes added to LSD to enhance the effect.

nationally, was going for $15 an ounce. LSD and mescaline started selling at $6 a tablet, but fell to $3 as competition drove down the price. The police had made an early decision to ignore drug use on the festival grounds.

Doctors and reporters who observed the scene estimated that 90 percent of festival-goers were high on marijuana and as many as half took some stronger drug.

Festival promoters knew from what had happened at other concerts that there would be many "bad trips" induced by LSD and other psychedelic drugs, ranging from anxiety attacks to temporary psychoses. They also expected some misuse of harder drugs like heroin and amphetamines. Alcohol would be thrown into the mix – a liquor store fifty miles from the site was sold out of wine on Friday night.

A freakout or bad trip was an unpleasant, sometimes horrific, reaction to a psychedelic drug, especially LSD. Researchers today suspect that LSD acts on serotonin receptors in the brain's cerebral cortex, which controls mood and thinking. They think the drug also affects the locus ceruleus, a brain area that processes sensory information.

Purple Haze

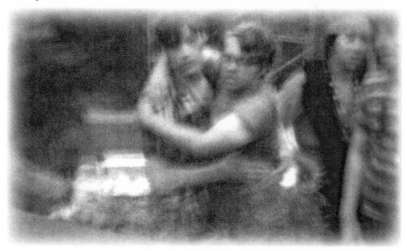

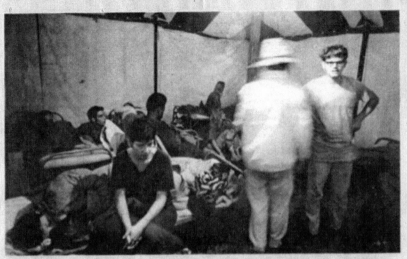

Temporary medical facilities, erected at the Hog Farm on the festival site, provides emergency treatment, primarily for those who "freaked out" on LSD.

The effects of acid were unpredictable and dependent on the user and the setting in which the drug was taken. Emotions were often intensified, with rapid swings from euphoria to paranoia. Colors, smells, sounds and other sensory input were intensified. Sometimes, the tripper saw sounds or felt colors. Hallucinations could be visual or could involve distortions of body image or time.

The effects of the drug were often so intense that the person suspected himself of going insane, dying, or being pursued by demons. Reassurance and a reminder that the acid will wear off were helpful in countering these symptoms.

Sometimes those undergoing a freakout somaticized their psychological stress, translating the experience into physical symptoms like stomach aches, heart palpitations, or nausea. This made diagnosis tricky – was the person physically ill or freaking out?

The press and some medical workers referred to LSD "overdoses" at Woodstock. "Bad reactions" is a more accurate term. What constitutes a lethal dose of LSD remains uncertain, but it's assumed to be many hundreds of times greater than the strongest street dose.

Experienced at treating LSD freakouts, Hog Farm members were often able to help the patient calm down enough so that no other intervention was called for. But the Farmers were also adept at recognizing the signs and symptoms of more serious drug problems. They quickly passed these cases on the doctors and nurses in the medical tent.

At first there was a good deal of skepticism on the part of both the Hog Farmers and their medical counterparts. But many of the doctors working at the festival were "hip" and understanding about youthful drug experimentation, and the medical people quickly came to see that the Hog Farm method was an effective way of dealing with freakouts.

Hog Farm leader Wavy Gravy noted the incongruity of the situation. Lacking some of his teeth at the time, and dressed in a cowboy hat that had belonged to Tom Mix with a rubber pig attached, his appearance was the antithesis of medical professionalism. "And I was supposed to tell these doctors what to do about crazy people."[25]

At the time, the standard treatment for LSD's mind-bending effects was Thorazine, a potent antipsychotic. The Hog Farmers opposed using Thorazine routinely – stopping a trip cold had negative psychological consequences, they felt. Doctors were willing to forgo the treatment, too. Thorazine had a number of potentially adverse side effects and interactions between the powerful tranquilizer and other drugs held the potential for unknown complications.

The Hog Farmers used a human, cognitive approach instead. They would touch patients, help them focus their minds on the present. They reassured them that they were experiencing the effects of a drug, not going crazy, and that those effects would wear off.

Many of those experiencing freakouts were young, away from home, lost in a crowd and subjected to trying conditions – mud, filth, noise, exposure, dehydration, too little sleep and too little food.

The Hog Farmers approached these people in just the right way, comforting them, making them feel part of a family, connected, and safe.

"It's rare when you can't come down off a bad trip and go into a good trip with help," asserted Hog Farmer Lisa Law.[26]

A description by Wavy Gravy of one of his encounters, as recounted in Joel Makower's *Woodstock: The Oral History*, gives a good snapshot of the Hog Farmers' method. The patient came into the medical tent in a highly agitated state. He was screaming, "Miami Beach, 1944!" and "Joyce! Joyce!" A number of doctors made ineffectual efforts to talk to him. Finally, Wavy approached the man.

> I said, "What's your name, man?" He says, "Joyce!" I said, "What's your name, man?" He says, "1944." I said, "WHAT'S YOUR NAME, MAN?" He says, "Bob." I said, "Your name is Bob!" And you could just see the Lost Hotels float out of his eyes. I said, "Your name is Bob. Your name is Bob. Your name is Bob." And he is getting it and he's getting it and he's getting it. And when he's got it I say, "Guess what?" He says, "What?" I said, "You took a little acid and it's going to wear off." He says, "Thank God."[27]

He goes on to explain that those who came down from their trips, usually after three or four hours, were encouraged to help others. Bob was told, "You see that sister coming through the door with her toes in her nose? That was you three hours ago. Now you're the doctor. Take over."

The method was simple, said one Hog Farmer, "Minister to them rather than do your trip on them."[28]

This relay method helped the original tripper to focus further and supplied manpower for the laborious task of talking down the hundreds in need of help. The Hog Farm had treated as many as 300 freakouts the first day and another 300 on Saturday.

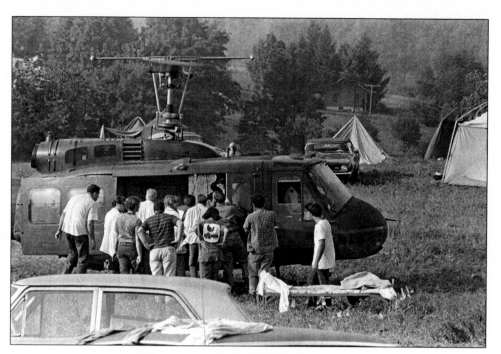

Getting airlifted out to the Rutherford School triage center

Wavy Gravy was not reluctant to turn over patients to the doctors when needed. One guy had taken "a Benzedrine factory" and would take days to talk down. Wavy recommended shooting him with injectable Valium. "If we told the doctors to give Valium they would," he said. "If we wanted to talk them down we talked them down. But only if it was doable."[29]

Some freakouts induced wild behavior. On Saturday night, a reporter observed a curly-headed blond boy being held down inside a panel truck.

"His eyes flashed wildly and he struggled with his would-be helpers. Inside a medical compound, the young man was held down by burly Liberty Ambulance Corps volunteers as hog farm leader Hugh Romney tried to 'talk him down.'

"The youth struggled violently with hog farmers and with the corpsmen holding his head, he was rushed to the main tent for treatment."[30]

Dr. Sydney Schiff treated a boy at the Rutherford School triage center who "was brought in in a markedly agitated state, actively hallucinating and in a panic. He described six men chasing him. I was told he had to be peeled off the underside of a bungalow where he was hiding in panic."[31]

Nurse Rikki Sanderson remembered treating a veteran from the Vietnam conflict, "He kept saying the same thing over and over again. He was afraid of something. 'Don't come near me,' he said. 'Don't come near me.' They tried to talk him down, but that time we did use drugs. They gave him a shot of something and an hour or so later he was down. We asked him, we always asked, what he had taken. I'm not awfully sure that we got the right answers."[32]

Sanderson had signed on to help at Woodstock not just for the $50 per diem wage but to learn more about treating drug cases. Her first patient, she remembered later, was a guy yelling "SPI-DERS!" She watched Hog Farm members treat the person with stroking and soft words.

"You learned in a gosh-darn fast way," she said. "You had to give them some touch with reality. You had to speak softly."[33]

Knowing the importance of a tranquil environment, the Hog Farmers made an effort to keep the freakout tent mellow. Wavy Gravy remembered blocking access to a cinematographer. "He wanted to go in and shoot inside the trip tent and I absolutely would not allow it."[34]

They recruited some of the headliners, including John Sebastian, to perform soothing music for the freakout victims. Jahanara, Wavy's wife, who went by the name Bonnie Jean Romney then, noted that "at one point when John Sebastian started to sing in the freakout tent, through my exhaustion and tiredness, it was like an angel had visited me. I remember I just began to weep with the beauty of it. . . . And the people who were writhing around and who were in pain, psychic pain, were just soothed."[35]

Sebastian remembers going to the medical tents with Rick Danko and singing, "Waiting for a Train" and "Stewball." He was struck by Wavy Gravy's ability to connect with those on bad trips.

"He would say, 'How much did you take, a hundred mikes [micrograms]? Well, I took a hundred last month and I know just what you're going through. We can get through this together.'"[36]

Abbie Hoffman had his own take in the drug problem. "You knew about the sugar and orange juice cure and Niacinamide tablets and Thorazine suppositories up the ass and when, as a last resort, to call a doctor," he said. There was anecdotal evidence that Niacinamide (vitamin B3) could reduce the effects of LSD. But Hoffman also pointed out the difficulty of diagnosis. The festival could be an awful place to trip, especially for first-time users. And since many drugs were bought from strangers, the user had no way of ascertaining the quality. "Was it strychnine or loss of ego?" Hoffman said. "Was it belladonna or the urban crisis?"[37]

These insights didn't stop the helpers from taking LSD themselves. When rumors of bad acid led fair-goers to turn over pills, Hog Farmers took them themselves because, as Wavy Gravy explained, "they were convinced it magnetized them to people that were having bum trips."[38]

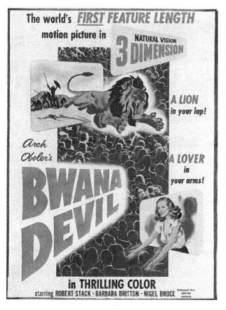

On Saturday evening Abbie Hoffman decided "to drop the second of the acid tabs people had been laying on me." The effects marked the end of Hoffman's volunteer medical role. "Things were becoming very unclear," he reported, "and when I saw a guy throw a spear at me like in the movie 'Bwana Devil' . . . I knew I was on some real powerful shit."[39] (Bwana Devil was the first 3-D feature, an African adventure film released in 1952).

65

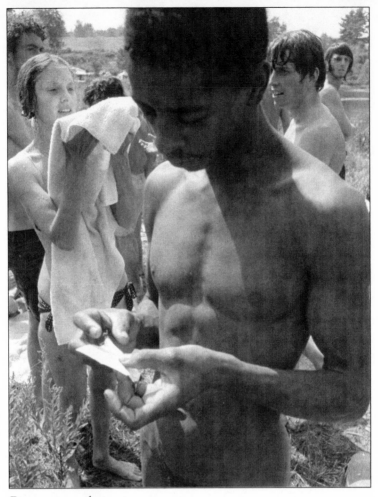

Drugs were prevalent

On Sunday, Woodstock Ventures promoter Artie Kornfeld, a vice president at Capital Records, became another drug casualty. He took a pill he thought was the mild stimulant Dexedrine, but that turned out to be psilocybin. "I was Thorazined out of it. That's why I missed Hendrix."[40]

On Sunday, Hendrix himself spent some time in the freakout tent dealing with his own purple haze. "We didn't know who he was," Nurse Sanderson said. "Just a black man lying on the stretcher. Then everybody started saying, 'Hey, isn't that Jimi Hendrix?' There was a big stir about it."[41]

The musician lay there for about 30 minutes before being corralled by his handlers. He had time to pull himself together as delays in the program meant that he didn't perform until Monday morning.

"It was chemical," one participant remembered. "Chemicals was where it was at. People were burning out left and right, big holes in the brain."[42]

The Hog Farmers and the medical people on duty at the festival formed a smooth working relationship. Jahanara was one of those responsible for the success of the collaboration. "The medical community surprised us," she said later. ". . . We began to see the value of the people there who were there medically trying to help, and vice versa. It got very nice."[43]

"We got our philosophy into the doctors' heads and they started treating people like we were treating people," remembered Hog Farmer Tom Law. "We knew how to deal with these kids because they were our generation."[44]

The Comanche and the Lawman

Deputy Sheriff Frank Zurawski was helping at the helicopter landing zone near the Rutherford School. He reported that a "hippie with hepatitis, and with what seemed to be a bad trip" refused to get off the chopper. The deputy removed him bodily, then talked him into seeing a doctor.

"As the doctor was talking to him, he started to carry on, saying 'I don't want to be with you people—I want to be with my own people. I don't want to see a doctor.'"

While he complained, the man was edging nearer to the door. "I attempted to hold him, and tried to calm him down, but he got more violent, and started to pull away from me. At that point the doctor told me to let him go. With that he took off like a 'Comanche' away from the school. Appropriately, he was dressed like an Indian."[45]

One of the controversies surrounding drug treatment was whether to try to warn festival-goers away from the drugs that seemed to be causing problems. On the one hand it might encourage them to seek early treatment. On the other hand, an announcement that the acid you had just taken was poison might in itself be enough to send users off on bad trips, even if the toxicity was a mere rumor.

Medicine for Trippers

Thorazine was the brand name of the drug chlorpromazine, the first specifically antipsychotic drug ever developed. When it appeared on the scene in the mid-1950s its effect was astounding – it emptied mental institutions of thousands of long-term patients. It was particularly effective in the treatment of schizophrenia. It gave hope to the hopeless.

Thorazine, one of a class of "major tranquilizers," was also indicated for the manic episodes of bipolar illness, and for anxiety, aggression, and amphetamine overdose. It seemed custom-made for reactions to LSD, which often made the tripper appear psychotic.

But the Hog Farmers probably had more insight into the situation than the doctors. Thorazine did have serious side effects. Slurred speech, lowering of seizure threshold, photosensitivity that could lead to sunburn, and low blood pressure were all possible.

Some critics called Thorazine a "chemical straitjacket." While it certainly dampened the hallucinations and paranoia of bad trips, the "talk down" method that the Hog Farmers used was effective, less dangerous, and better for the patient's long-term well-being.

The more commonly used treatment for freakouts at Woodstock was liquid Valium, the brand name of the drug diazepam, which was given in intramuscular and intravenous injections. Valium had been developed by the Swiss company Hoffman-La Roche in 1963 and had become wildly popular in the 1960s. It was the first billion-dollar drug, and by 1969 was the most prescribed medication in the world.

Valium was a "minor tranquilizer," for treatment of anxiety rather than psychosis. It was considered safer than the barbiturates it replaced for many uses, including insomnia, and epilepsy. It had few serious side effects when used therapeutically other than drowsiness and amnesia – many of those who slept off their trips under the influence of Valium at the Rutherford school awoke not knowing how they'd gotten there.

Some announcements were made from the stage about "bad acid." Since there were all kinds of acid in all kinds of colors, the warning was largely meaningless. The consensus is that there was probably little or no poison being sold as drugs, that some of the acid might have been badly manufactured, but that most bad trips had their origins in setting and psyche. "If you're worried," one announcement advised, "just take half a tablet."[46]

In any case, the Hog Farmers and the medical personnel both had their work cut out for them. "I cannot overemphasize how hard we were working," Jahanara said. "There was almost no possibility of sleep."[47]

Survive and Share

By Saturday, coping with adversity became a subtext of the whole festival. Sometime on Saturday, Abbie Hoffman and his colleagues put out a leaflet headed "**SURVIVE SURVIVE SURVIVE**." Excerpts give a flavor of the mood that suffused Woodstock as the festival moved through its second trying day:

> Welcome to Hip City, USA. We're now one of the largest cities in America (population 300,000 and growing all the time....This is a disaster area...
>
> Where we go from here depends on all of us. The people who promoted the festival have been overwhelmed by their own creation. We can no longer remain passive consumers; we have to fend for ourselves....
>
> A planeload of doctors are being airlifted from New York City and a fleet of helicopters is being gathered to drop medical supplies. Any trained medical personnel around report to the.... medical centers.

Do not take any light blue flat acid and understand
that taking strong dope at this time may make you
a drag in a survival situation....

You should not be piggish about your food and water.
As with medicine, festival people have promised
that food will be airlifted into the area....

The thing to do is survive and share. Organize
your own camping area so that everyone makes it
through uncomfortable times ahead. Figure out what
you must do and the best ways to get it done.[48]

Water, Water, Everywhere

Two aspects of the festival related to health care were the availability of clean drinking water and the disposal of human waste. Both were a source of concern beforehand and both were cited as problem afterward. But while all did not go smoothly in either case, neither contributed significant health issues.

The concern was justified by the fact that the rural area where the festival was to be held had neither a municipal water supply nor any facilities for handling sewage. All water and sanitation had to be arranged from scratch for the festival.

Woodstock Ventures people worked with engineers from the New York State Department of Health to plan the water supply. They pumped water from a nearby lake and ran it through sand and gravel swimming pool filters, then chlorinated it. This system could furnish 259,000 gallons a day. The water was stored in four 12,000 gallon tanks and distributed to the site through a system of pipes.

Four 300-foot-deep wells in the campground area also supplied a spigot system there to provide water for cooking, washing and drinking. This water was also chlorinated. Because festival-goers camped in areas beyond the designated campground, promoters

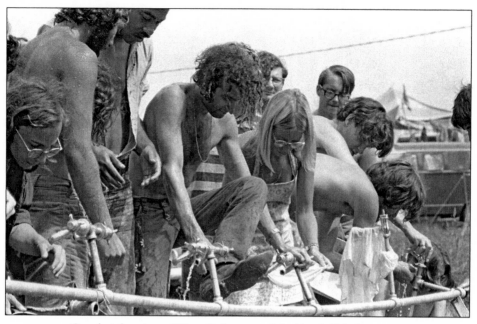

Crowd at the spigots. Who said there weren't bathing facilities?

used five converted milk trucks, each holding 5,800 gallons, to provide supplies in more remote parts of the site.

The tanks that supplied the main system were never less than a quarter full, even at the time of highest usage. Some mains and spigots broke, but problems were quickly addressed and flow restored.

Some local residents took advantage of the need and sold water to thirsty festival-goers. When Max Yasgur heard about this, he was furious. "How can anyone ask money for water?" he wanted to know. Soon his barn bore a large sign announcing, "Free Water."[49]

One factor that helped conserve water was the heavy chlorination that state protocols called for. Though the water was safe, it was not particularly palatable. "Many of the campers were organic and objected to the chlorination of water," a state health official reported.[50] This held down demand for drinking water.

Sanitation was a different story. Festival organizers had a hard time pinning down exactly how many toilets were appropriate for the crowd of 50,000 originally expected. They ended up contracting with the New York City company, Johnny-On-The-Spot, Corporation, for 30 portable chemical toilets known as Big John units. Each had ten stalls and five urinals and a 900-gallon tank. Port-O-San out of Kearny, New Jersey, provided 250 single units, for a total of 550 toilets seats. Though a state health inspector judged this to be "plenty," it was woefully inadequate for the huge crowd.[51]

As early as Saturday morning, Woodstock Ventures operations director Mel Lawrence found the toilets near concession area "in real bad shape . . . they were filthy and disgusting."[52] The problem was overuse and the difficulty of getting trucks in to pump the units out. The toilets were soon overflowing.

Though the units were near roads, moving trucks around the festival grounds became increasingly difficult. Because of abandoned cars, getting out to the dumping site three miles away was also slow going. The decision was made to dig an eighty-foot long trench, eight feet deep, in a remote part of the grounds and dump some of

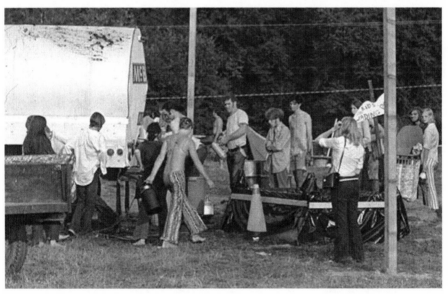

One of five 5,800-gallon converted milk trucks sent to areas lacking piped water

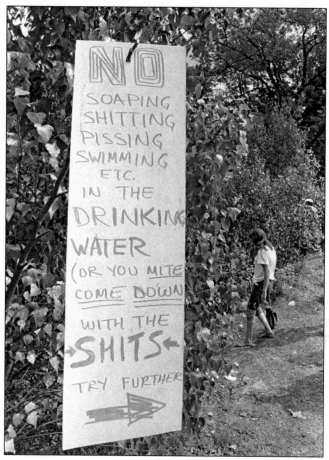

The Department of Health could not have said it better

the sewage there. Though workers laced it heavily with chemicals and covered it, the stench was unavoidable.

Long lines and putrid toilets induced some fair-goers to make use of corn fields and the back yards of neighboring homes to relieve themselves. They sought out gas stations and restaurants in order to make use of their facilities.

"There was a shortage of bathrooms" said fair-goer Liz Fulton, "but there was no shortage of bushes."[53]

Health inspectors at the festival faced a sometimes trying task. Martin J. Cohen was a junior high school science teacher who had

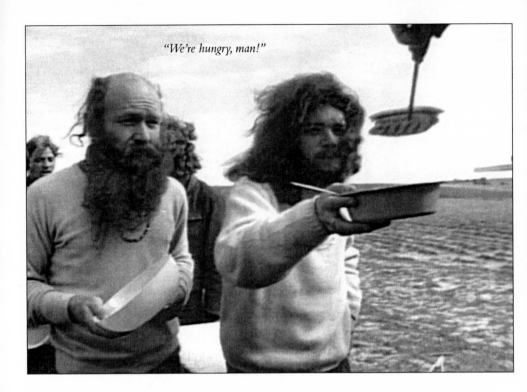
"We're hungry, man!"

taken a summer job as an inspector for the New York State Health
Department's Monticello district office. On Friday afternoon, he
volunteered to work overtime overseeing food, water, and sanitation
facilities at the festival.

"I had a crewcut, white shirt, black pants, [and] a clip board . . .
My first vender was dressed with a cook's hat, love beads, shoulder
length hair, beard, earrings, cowboy boots and a loin cloth. He
was selling grilled hamburgers. I sternly admonished him that he
was in violation of many basic health codes, unsafe food handling,
possible pubic hairs in the food, and that he should stop selling
the hamburgers until he cleaned up these violations. A crowd of
'Hippies' began to gather around us, shouting, 'We're hungry man,
get lost!' He said, 'You know where you can put that clipboard.' It
became instantly clear to me that my safety depended on a quick
retreat, mumbling to my self, "What am I am doing here?"[54]

Garbage also became a serious problem. In the middle of his performance Arlo Guthrie made a plea to the crowd, "please throw your garbage on the road." Guthrie was serious. He was asked by maintenance men to explain that garbage on the road was easier to clean up than garbage strewn about the fields.[55]

Huge amounts of trash piled up during the festival, and mountains of it were left behind. But, as one inspector observed, while it looked bad, it was for the most part not organic and presented no health threat.

We Were Half a Million Strong

How many attended the Woodstock Festival?

The answer will always involve guesswork. On Saturday, New York State Police Maj. John Monahan guessed that 400,000 were at the site. Some said that by Sunday the crowd had reached 450,000. Some said 480,000. That figure, conveniently rounded to 500,000, was made famous when Joni Mitchell, in her anthem "Woodstock," declared "we were half a million strong."

Al Romm, then editor of the *Times Herald-Record* in Middletown, insisted the crowd was much smaller. He said aerial photos show only 150,000. But Bert Feldman, Bethel town historian, held that the fair attracted an even larger crowd than was reported. "There were 700,000 people there," he said. "The attendance estimate is based on aerial photos and there were thousands of people under trees."[17]

The fluid nature of the crowd adds another uncertainty. Many came late, many left early. All that can be said with certainty is that it was the largest rock and roll festival and the largest gathering of young people in history up to that time.

EXTRA
EXTRA
The Times Herald RECORD
400,000 flood site; rock crisis eases off
Full report, Pages 2-9

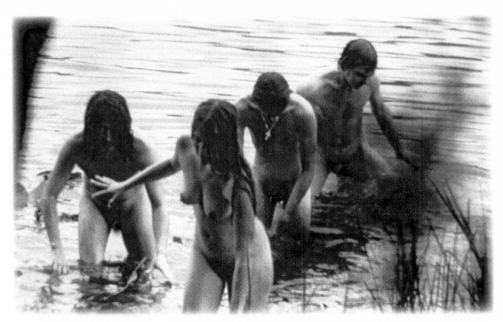

Some of the bathing was for pleasure, some for cleanliness. But almost all of it was nude.

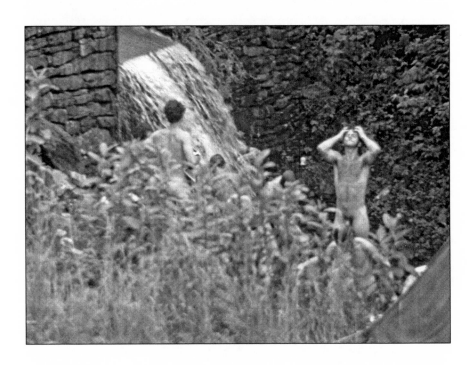

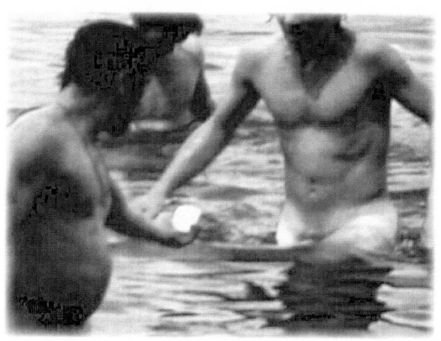

Sharing the soap (a still from a super 8 mm film)

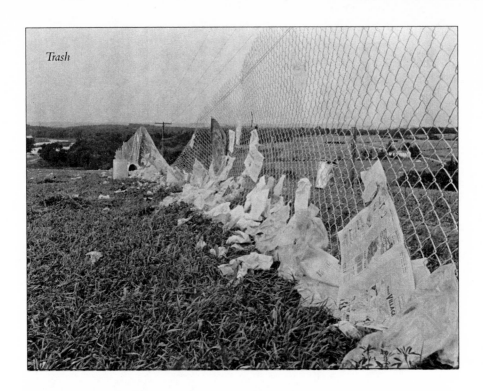

Trash

Monitoring public health and sanitation at the festival was Gerald Lieber, who headed the Monticello Sub-District Office of the New York State Department of Health. Lieber led a staff of approximately a dozen inspectors and sanitary engineers whose usual summer duties were to inspect camps and bungalow colonies in the resort area. He minimized problems at the festival in his report, and laid those that did arise to visitors who camped in unauthorized "squatter sectors" that were "not furnished with water, toilet facilities or refuse containers." [56]

"All of our health facilities were really taxed, but they were working," said Mel Lawrence. "This man came down and he was going to inspect everything and hold us to the letter of the law of sanitation. I knew if he did this, we were going to get popped." [57]

Richard Mattox was the Health Department planning consultant from Albany whom Lawrence referred to. He was assigned to keep an eye on sanitation, but he spent much of his time at the festival

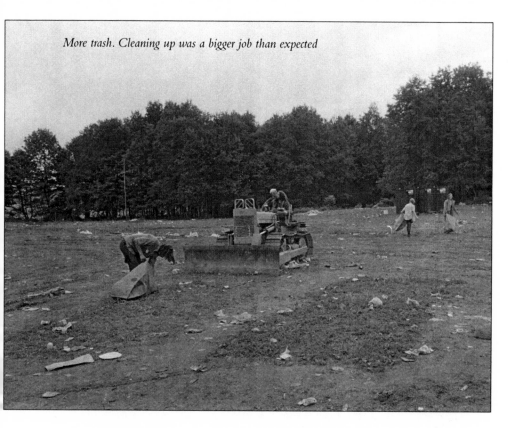
More trash. Cleaning up was a bigger job than expected

hunting for his teenage daughter, who had come with him but gotten separated.

"I think a very real effort was made under some very real handicaps, such as the rain and the size of the crowds," Mattox said afterward. "A satisfactory job was done. Water supplies were, as far as I could observe, adequate."[58]

Much was made afterward of the nude bathing that went on at the festival. In fact, no arrangements had been made to provide showers for fair-goers. Because of the pervasive mud, filth and heat, many took advantage of the chance to clean off offered by nearby lakes and ponds.

Sheriff Ratner observed, "You must remember that many of these youths were in the mud, that they had been in the rain for several hours and that they had to get clean."[59]

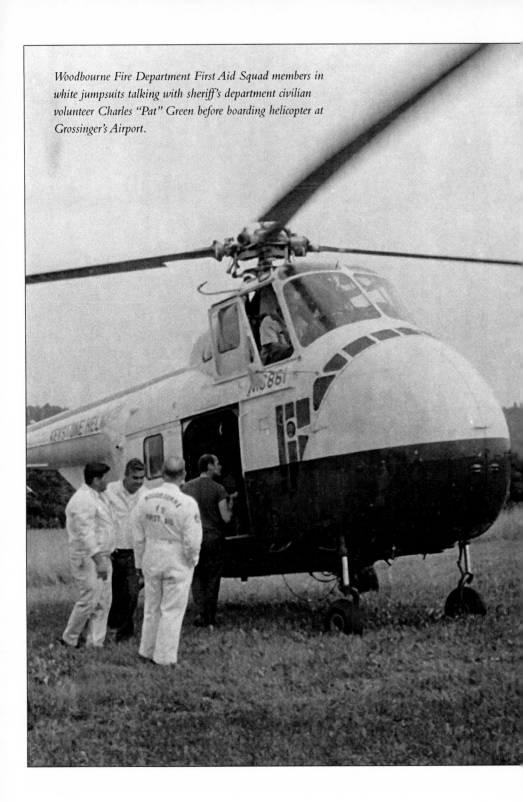

Woodbourne Fire Department First Aid Squad members in white jumpsuits talking with sheriff's department civilian volunteer Charles "Pat" Green before boarding helicopter at Grossinger's Airport.

3

~~~~~~~~~~~~~~~~~~~~~~~

Health and Healing

GLEN JOSHPE had spent many childhood summers in White Lake, a hamlet in the town of Bethel. In August 1969 he was an intern at New York Medical College in Manhattan and was returning to visit his parents at their bungalow. His mother called him Wednesday night and said to come up early, a stampede was expected the next day.

Joshpe arrived and found his father renting out lawn space to festival-goers for $5 a tent. He headed over to the festival grounds himself to enjoy some music. Curious about the medical facilities, he walked over to the medical tent. He ran into Dr. Abruzzi, who was asking, "Does anyone have any IV Valium?" A patient was having a seizure.

Joshpe volunteered that he had Valium in his medical kit back at his family bungalow. The next thing he knew, he was on a helicopter, touching down outside the cottage. He sprinted past his shocked parents, grabbed his bag, and headed back to the site.

The patient flow in the medical tent was, to Joshpe, similar to that in a large urban emergency room. It was typical to find thirty or forty patients lying on gurneys, half with medical problems, half with drug-induced crises.

"Many had forgotten their medicines from home or lost their medicines or left them in the car," he wrote in his memoir *Joshpe's Journey.* "There were a number of diabetics who needed insulin, and the usual amounts of colds, sore throats, fevers, and other problems that you would expect to see in any city the size of Buffalo."

To bring order to the tent, he recommended separating those who had been seen from those who were awaiting examination.

"Many of the treatments," Joshpe remembered, "had to be improvised, such as the treating of a case of Digitalis toxicity with orange juice, since we had no potassium."

Joshpe was impressed by the treatment that Hog Farm members provided to patients having bad reactions to drugs. He remembered them forming a large circle around a campfire, with the most acute cases in the center. Patients moved outward as they calmed down.

"Their approach was revolutionary and carried significantly less risk than heavily sedating a patient . . . who was already severely intoxicated."

The Hog Farmers kept patients talking, gave them coffee and donuts, explained that their hallucinations weren't real. "Within an hour, the acute became sub-acute, and before long they were helping others. It was only rarely that the physicians needed to intervene with drugs."

Like many other volunteers, Joshpe has fond memories of his experience. "Doctors, nurses, and medical students would come and go and take breaks, enjoy the music. It was one of the most exciting, enjoyable three days of my life."[1]

When Woodstock Ventures handed over the $25,000 that the organization had agreed to donate to the town where the festival was held, officials decided to use it to build a clinic known as the Bethel Medical Center. Joshpe, who helped equip the center and served as its first physician, became known as the Woodstock Doc.

One Patient's Story

Robert Flynn lived in North Branch, New York, in 1969, only 16 miles from Bethel. He went to the festival on Tuesday with ten friends and set up a large tent. While getting dressed on Saturday morning, he struck his eye on a brass belt buckle hanging from the tent post. Thinking nothing the matter and "dropping a hit of mescaline," he headed down to the pond for a morning dip.

"As time passed, the pain in my eye became worse and worse." He tried to rest but the pain only increased. "We headed to the medical tent round 1:30-2:00 Sunday morning. . . . I don't recall a waiting line and saw a doctor quickly. I remember him putting some amber colored liquid in my eye and examining me with the usual hand held magnifying light thing. He determined that I had severely scratched my cornea, and that with the filthy and unsanitary conditions all around, suggested that I leave the festival, or risk infection and possible loss of the eye."

The doctor cleaned the wound, applied salve and a patch, and Flynn departed. He and his friends knew the back roads and had no trouble getting home. His mother took him to a doctor that same day, and he was admitted to the hospital in Liberty.

A nurse drove Flynn to the festival site on Tuesday to retrieve his tent and other belongings. Accompanying them was young man suffering from multiple sclerosis, a long-term patient at the hospital, who had been following the action at Woodstock on a short-wave radio. Flynn's new companion was astounded to see the reality of the festival grounds.[2]

The Nurses

Among the unsung heroes of the Woodstock Festival were the nurses who pitched in to provide care. Some were hired, some volunteered. Much of the medical care required was within the nurses' realm: cleaning and dressing small wounds, giving tetanus shots, establishing intravenous lines, and providing comfort and support. One of their key duties was triage, quickly evaluating incoming patients and deciding which ones needed urgent treatment, which needed to be transported to hospitals, which were lower priority. They worked long hours on little sleep processing the endless lines of festival-goers in distress.

Rikki Sanderson was a registered nurse who ran a preschool in Middletown and had two teenagers of her own. She had been hired in advance by Woodstock Ventures to work a couple of shifts at the fair. When the crowds mushroomed, promoters asked her to recruit as many other nurses as she could, and she passed on the word to colleagues.

When she entered the pink medical tent Saturday afternoon, Sanderson saw "a mass of bodies on the floor. Some were on low cots, some with intravenous tubes, some huddled up, some sleeping. "The facilities in the tent were basic. There was only one IV pole among the bare cots."[3]

Sanderson was shocked when Dr. Abruzzi told her she was in charge of the tent. "I had

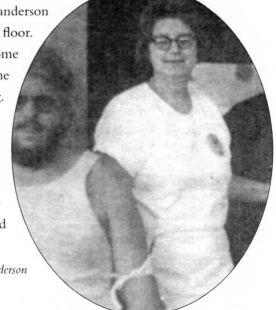

Rikki Sanderson

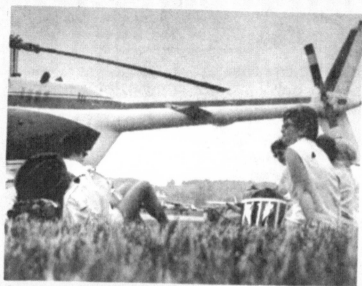

Four nurses from Middletown area await helicopter trip to Yasgur Farms site of Aquarian Exposition. The ladies, all volunteers, were part of large medical staff called in to aid ill "festivalians."   *--TH-Record photo by Jay Lange*

only gone to help," she said, but duty called and she began to work on the steady stream of patients. "Their feet were cut to ribbons," she remembered. She had them put their feet in bowls of clean water and disinfectant before further cleaning the wounds.[4]

Abruzzi introduced her to Diane from the Hog Farm and left. Diane, "a very young, very beautiful, very clean girl," gave her a quick rundown about the drugs that people were taking and how to treat overdosed patients.

"When a patient came in, we asked what color pill and how many," Sanderson told a reporter. "You must ask very kindly. The youngster mustn't think you're interrogating him or he won't come back."

Many patients did not want to give their names. "One young man said if his parents knew he was at Woodstock, they would ground him for life or worse," another nurse remembered.[5]

Many nurses reported a relentless stream of patients, but the pattern of injuries varied and some were far from overwhelmed. Barbara Crispell (now Wexler) was a staff nurse at Liberty Hospital who flew in from Grossinger's Airport. "But as big a deal as that was, I really didn't do very much, kind of sat around waiting for people to come, and passed out tampons and band aids. At one pont we thought there was going to be a delivery and got that all set up – my background was labor and delivery -- but there was no delivery, at least while I was there."[6]

An Amazing Sight

Many of the nurses were amazed by the scene they encountered at the festival. Lucille Thalmann (now Rudiger), who worked as a nurse at the hospital in Liberty, had planned to go to the festival to celebrate her eleventh wedding anniversary. She heard about the problems and "decided to get to the site and volunteer my services." A native of the area, she was able to navigate back roads into the site.

"I was astonished at the sights and sounds I encountered," she remembered later. "It was surreal, as if I stepped into another world. Loud music, rain, nudity, profanity, open fornication, the smell of marijuana floating over the entire site...I certainly won't forget it."[7]

Patients streamed into the tent through the night. To Sanderson, the music blaring from the stage lent the scene a "nightmarish" quality.[8]

Frances Marks was one of the ones who responded to the need that was becoming apparent on Friday. With her friend and fellow nurse Beatrice Pollets she went to the Orange County Airport in Montgomery, but they were bumped from the five-place helicopter by Doctors Sutton and Herrera and their medical equipment. Instead, a police car showed up to take them over the clogged roads and into the site.

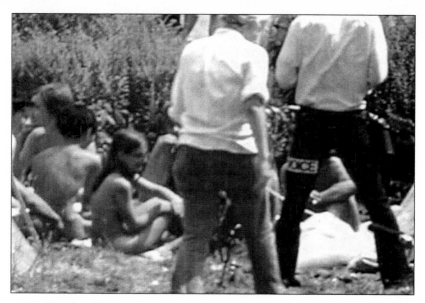

Casual nudity was common

Another who responded knew the territory better than any of them. She was Lois Yasgur, daughter of the farmer on whose land the festival was held. A registered nurse in New York, she and her husband came to Bethel for the festival but never reached her parents' home. After walking several miles, they reached the site and found that medical help was needed. Her mother, Miriam, remembered that "she went into the hospital tent and worked there and then went home. I never saw her."[9]

Barbara Hahn, who lived only a few miles from the Yasgur farm, came in on Saturday. She was a volunteer dispatcher with the Jeffersonville Volunteer Ambulance Corps, which operated in the town just north of Bethel, and a registered nurse. Her husband was a veterinarian.

On Saturday afternoon she heard that calls had gone out for volunteers and she drove over to the airport at Grossinger's Resort Hotel for a helicopter flight into the grounds. She found about a dozen people at Grossinger's, including Edyth Hyatt, a retired Army nurse who had worked in a field hospital in Italy, and Dr.

Lee Tompkins, the public health officer of the Town of Liberty. Informed that antibiotics were in short supply, Hahn had brought along a supply of human-label tetracycline that her husband used in his practice to treat calf diarrhea. Each bottle had 1,000 capsules.

Ruth Aprilante was called by another nurse and asked to work. She was told to wear her white uniform. A police helicopter picked her up in Fosterdale, five miles west of Bethel, and flew her in.

"I was frozen in sheer terror as I do not like to fly," she remembered. But over the site her fear changed to amazement. "I could not believe what I saw."[10]

Barbara Hahn was also awed by the masses of people. Walking through the crowd with Dr. Tompkins, she asked him to hold her hand. "I was frightened."

But she pitched in and went to work. "My first patient dove into shallow water and split his head open," she recalled. "I asked, 'Are you still tripping?' and he said, 'The trip is over.'"[11]

For a time Tompkins took over Big Pink, the circus tent that housed the field hospital, while Dr. Abruzzi maintained overall command. "Dr. Abruzzi was in charge and seemed to do a good job," Hahn said. "There were really no problems, many volunteers just walked in from the audience and offered to help."[12]

Frances Marks said an area of the tent was curtained off so that doctors and nurses could grab a nap now and then. "I'd go over there at two or three in the morning and all of a sudden you'd hear screaming and you'd have to get up. So I barely got an hour or two of sleep the three nights."[13]

Marks's friend Beatrice Pollets worked in the first aid trailer with Dr. Abruzzi. "Whenever I would go out to get a fresh breath of air," she reported, "I'd come back in and couldn't stop smiling."[14]

She asked Abruzzi why she was smiling even though she was so tired. He told her she was stoned, not because she had touched drugs, but because the air was so perfumed with marijuana smoke.

"I just had to breathe and got stoned," she said. She might also have been experiencing a "contact high," in which the euphoric feelings of the stoned fair-goers became contagious.

The main injuries she saw were cut feet. Patients were sutured, given a tetanus shot, and in most cases those who had footwear "put on their sandals and away they went."

Long lines formed outside the medical trailer. The nurses were advised to be careful with supplies, though no serious shortages ever developed.

Frances Marks helped treat some kids high on drugs who had had an encounter with the barbed wire that was used for fencing in part of the farm. They came in with lacerations to their arms and the doctor gave them medication to calm them if needed and "we would sit there and talk to the kids and hold their hands."

She remembered medications, including tranquilizers, being

Lethal Pop Tops

I blew out my flip flop,
Stepped on a pop top,
Cut my heel, had to cruise on back home.

So Jimmy Buffett sang in his 1977 song "Margaritaville." The first detachable opener arrived in 1963 on cans holding Iron City Beer. Schlitz took the idea national two year later. All you had to do was grab a ring and pull. A little strip of attached metal came off and your can was open. By the time of the Woodstock festival, the pop top was standard on all beer and soda cans.

Pop tops were handy. They obviated the need for a church key, the common name for a pointed can opener used to pierce holes in the tops of beer cans. But pop tops were also an environmental nightmare. Most people tossed them on the ground, where they became hazardous litter. They were replaced in the mid-1970s with the stay tabs familiar today.

No accounting was kept at Woodstock of the source of cut feet, but certainly pop tops contributed their share, along with broken glass and jagged rocks. Hidden in the mud, those sharp curls could offer a nasty surprise to barefoot concert-goers.

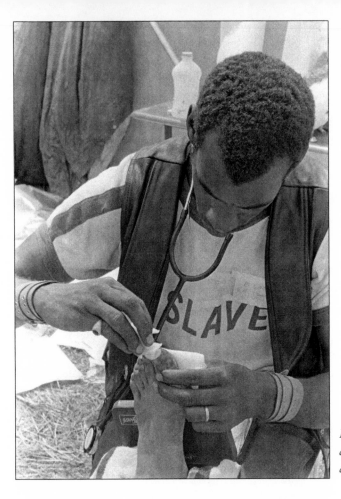

Helping —
and making
a statement

injected intramuscularly or intravenously. Many of the patients she saw were thirsty, as fresh water wasn't always readily available. They would be given a drink and something to eat.

Barbara Hahn learned that getting a drug patient to move his tongue was a good idea. When an ambulance attendant radioed that they had a boy who had collapsed from a bad trip, "I told them to have him wiggle his tongue and he was fine – not fine but he didn't need an ambulance."

She also remembered an ophthalmologist from Canada who was following rock festivals all summer to study the effect of drugs on the eye. "He came in with his ophthalmoscope and looked at people's eyes."

There was talk of setting aside part of the tent for those LSD users who had damaged their eyes staring at the sun. Rumors of this danger circulated widely at the time but proved to be mythical.

John Pinnavaia, an 18-year-old from Brooklyn, stepped on a broken bottle in the mud on Sunday night. He didn't realize how badly he'd been cut until a girl nearby started screaming.

"This guy picked me up, threw me over his shoulder and ran me to the hospital," he remembered later. "Must have saved my life."

From the medical tent a helicopter flew him to Monticello Hospital, where doctors stitched a deep cut. They called his home to ask permission for the procedure. "Mom freaked out."

Pinnavaia spent four months on crutches, but the injury had a silver lining. Before he went to Woodstock, he had been classified 1-A, ready for service, by his draft board. His injury earned him a 1-Y, a temporary disability rating. He then married, lowering himself further on the list. His "Woodstock Wound" helped keep him out of the jungles of Vietnam.[15]

I Will Never Forget

A doctor diagnosed one girl as suffering from a ruptured appendix. He wanted to send her out to a hospital, but she was with another girl and would not go without her friend. In spite of the potential severity of her illness, she wouldn't leave her companion, even though they had met only a few hours earlier. "Those two girls went off and we never knew what happened to her, just turned and went off. It was peace and love," said Beatrice Pollets.

Frances Marks's husband Ansel was a urologist working at Horton Hospital in Middletown during the festival. He treated one case of renal failure. Because no dialysis machine was available, he used the method known as peritoneal dialysis, which involved

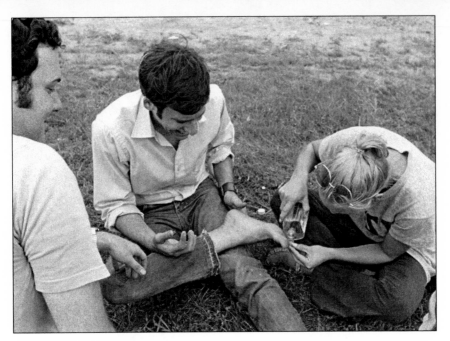

Ouch!

injecting fluid into the patient's abdominal cavity, where it collects waste products from the blood before being drained.

Dr. Marks also catheterized some patients from the festival. "Some went into retention because of overload and some because of the drugs they were taking."

Rose Raimond, the evening charge nurse at Monticello Hospital was not as sanguine as others working through the long weekend. "It was the worst day of my life," she reported. "We couldn't leave."

Patients never stopped coming in. "They ate us out of everything, we didn't have enough food to feed our [other] patients."[16]

Back at the site, nurse Ruth Aprilante was impressed by the treatment the Hog Farmers gave to the drug cases. They "would come and take these kids on trips and stay with them until they were better. They had set up a quiet area with sleeping bags/mattresses not far from the medical trailers."

Barbara Hahn agreed. She observed Wavy Gravy talk a kid down from a trip. "It was educational. I had no experience with it before."

Hahn emphasized how critical it was that the wounded fair-goers were routinely given tetanus shots. "A short time afterward, my husband was called to the Yasgur farm to look at a sick cow and it had tetanus. It wasn't common, but it did happen on farms, so it was important the kids got their shots."

Many of the nurses found the experience at Woodstock a memorable one. "It was exciting," Fran Marks remembered.

Rikki Sanderson had to go home at 10:30 Monday morning. "I just had to get out of there for a little while . . . close my mind a little." She returned Monday afternoon and found 50 patients in the medical tent. "Without exception their feet were all cut to pieces."[18]

Nurse Pollets found kids very grateful for the help they received and later stated, "I enjoyed it even though it was totally exhausting. It was a wonderful experience for me, one of the highlights of my life."

She even found that her experience there had a significant effect on her strained relationship with her son. "When he found out I went there to help kids, he treated me differently. From then on we got along very well."

"Woodstock," said Ruth Aprilante, "I will never forget."

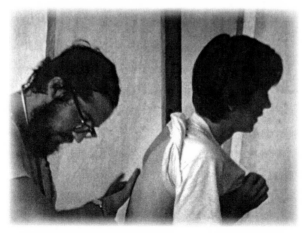

A "hip doctor" helps out

Airlift

The road to Woodstock from New York City included 48 miles on the New York State Thruway and another 45 miles along four-lane Route 17, known as the Quickway. The last ten miles followed a local road, Route 17B. By Saturday, 17B was virtually impassible because of the traffic and abandoned cars. Route 17 was also seriously clogged. Moving patients out of the festival site and supplies and personnel in had become a serious logistical problem.

Fortunately, the promoters had contracted with a fleet of helicopters, including small two-seat and medium five-seat choppers and larger twelve-seaters. Part of their duty was to ferry entertainers from the airport at Grossinger's Resort Hotel to the area behind the main stage. These choppers were also assigned to bring in the supplies that would sustain the rock celebrities, including pâté and champagne. Such indulgences enraged Abbie Hoffman, who tossed off cases of bubbly to make room for needed medical supplies.

It soon became clear that these helicopters were not going to be sufficient. On Saturday morning, Sheriff Ratner put out the word that additional help was needed and a message of *Immediate* precedence was sent up the military chain of command. Approval for the use of Army helicopters came down from Aerospace Command Headquarters in Colorado Springs and from the Pentagon.

Air Force Reserve Colonel Leif Halvorsen was serving as the Air Force Disaster Preparedness Officer for the state at the time. He was told "a health disaster was pending, and assistance was requested."

Halvorsen arranged for two Army UH-1D Huey helicopters to be sent from Stewart Air Force Base, about fifty miles from the site. The larger choppers, part of 102nd Aviation Assault Helicopter Command, were usually stationed in Fort Bragg, NC. That summer they were at Stewart to support the training of cadets at West Point, about 15 miles away. The unit was commanded by Captain Bobby L Blake, a Vietnam veteran.

These Huey choppers were a familiar sight to anyone who watched the news those days, as they were used extensively in the raging Vietnam war. They could hold twelve people in addition to the two-man crew, and fly at 120 miles an hour. They had room for six stretchers.

The Army had the helicopters, but no medical personnel to man them. Recruited from Stewart to providing this expertise were Air Force Captain and physician Dennis Glazer and three medics. Soon after touching down at the festival, Glazer found that his young assistants had wandered off. They soon returned, having been sorely tempted by the non-medical aspects of the festival.

After being activated at 4:15 p.m. Saturday afternoon, the Army choppers flew out 97 patients in a little more than 24 hours. They brought in 2500 pounds of food.

Colonel Halvorsen remembered landing near the hospital tent and removing kids who had overdosed. In spite of the anti-military

This helicopter is a U.S. Army UH-1D Huey, not an Air Force helicopter

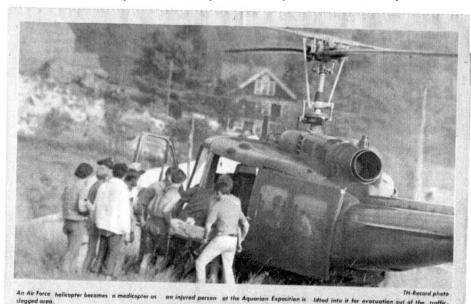

An Air Force helicopter becomes a medicopter as an injured person at the Aquarian Exposition is lifted into it for evacuation out of the traffic-slogged area.

TH-Record photo

feelings prevalent among the Woodstock generation, he said, "All of a sudden, we weren't the bad guys."[19]

News reports and other accounts would later assert that the National Guard was activated to provide this airlift capability. But although New York State officials contemplated using the Guard, units were never called up. The military helicopters that would serve Woodstock were provided by the regular Army and manned by Air Force medical personnel.

"The helicopters flew in and out of the Rutherford site," remembered Monticello school superintendent Charles Rudiger, "bringing in stoned kids and some with broken bones and lacerations, and flying back with hard-boiled eggs, sandwiches, bottled soda."[20]

" Announcement From the Stage

Somebody may have noticed or all of you may have noticed a familiar-colored helicopter over there. The United States Army has lent us some medical teams and is giving us a hand. They're with us man, not against us. They are with us. They are here to give us all a hand and help us and for that they deserve it. "

Sheriff deputies at the school put up a wind sock to guide pilots, kept the zone clear, and formed two lines of men to load the supplies that were flown in by the returning helicopters. They also prevented hippies anxious to get back to the festival from climbing onto the choppers. At one point, Blake grounded his helicopters briefly when they became a taxi service. "We're here on a humanitarian mission to bring out the sick and bring in supplies," the Captain told local officials.[21]

The regular arrival and departure of helicopters annoyed some spectators and musicians, but the pilots did a superb job under trying circumstances. Many of them were veterans of the Vietnam jungles and, as one observer noted, "This was a piece of cake to them."[22]

As Monticello hospital president Gordon Winarick admitted, the system of evacuating patients from the festival "just kind of evolved." Yet it worked well. It saved the life of at least one person suffering a serious drug overdose and took pressure off of the overworked medical people at the festival site.

Disaster Averted

When Woodstock Ventures promoter Joel Rosenman phoned the medical group late Saturday afternoon, they said they were still short-handed. He went out to check and possibly round up more volunteers. But when he reached the field hospital "the condition of medical services appeared to be excellent. There were a good many first aid cases wandering about, but treatment seemed to be more prompt here than in most New York City hospitals."[23]

"Everything came together," noted Winarick. "It was an outpouring. Everybody did what was right."[24]

Dr. Abruzzi remained in charge of the medical effort at Woodstock throughout. "Abruzzi was so calm and confident that everyone was amazed," said one observer.[25]

Certainly, Abruzzi could not have done it alone. Initially hesitant about using volunteers, he clearly had no choice after the festival crowd began to swell. Scores of doctors and nurses responded to the call for volunteers. Some were already at the festival. Others came from local communities, others from New York City. Dr. Seymour Cohen of Monticello was among the local doctors who knew the back roads and managed to make their way into the festival and out again, covering shifts and going home to rest.

Patients who needed urgent care were airlifted directly to Monticello Hospital, a ten-mile hop. This was a time when

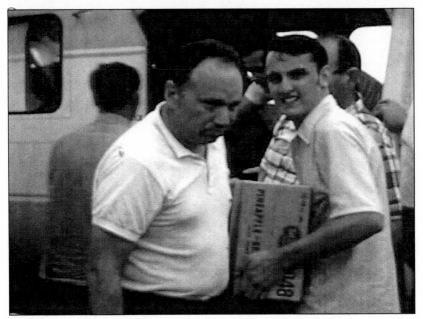

Eighteen-year-old Monticello volunteer Howard Perlman (right) helps load helicopter with food supplies at the Rutherford School

emergency transport by helicopter was rare in civilian emergencies. Most hospitals, including Monticello, lacked dedicated landing zones. But in the emergency officials made a swift decision for the choppers to bring in patients.

Mischa Leshner, Monticello Hospital administrator, allowed small helicopters to land on the hospital's flat roof. "If it could hold all those snow accumulations in the winter, it should be able to support a helicopter," he reasoned.[26] Later, space was cleared in the hospital's parking lot to allow for larger helicopters to land.

The majority of festival patients who needed further care were airlifted to the Rutherford Elementary School triage center in Monticello. A regular infirmary was established there in order to free up the hospitals for more serious emergencies. The gymnasium held about 150 cots and became a ward for the tired and less seriously ill. More acute cases were handled in the auditorium, where some patients were given intravenous fluids.

Originally, the school was to have been used to bivouac National Guard troops who might be activated in the event of a full-scale riot. Helen Reno, a community volunteer at the facility, remembered that Woodstockers were routinely led to the showers where aides helped clean them of mud before they were allowed into the gym to be examined.[27]

The school was manned at first by volunteer doctors who happened to be in the area. Dr. Sydney Schiff, who was in charge, gradually replaced them with local doctors whose skills he knew. This location became central in coordinating patient flow and sending medical and food supplies into the festival. By Saturday

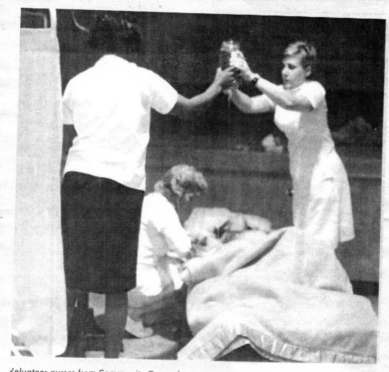

Volunteer nurses from Community General Hospital administer emergency treatment to one of many young men and women affected by drug freak-outs. Treatment was given in an emergency hospital set up in Kenneth L. Rutherford Elementary School in Monticello

--TH-Record photo by Charlie Crist

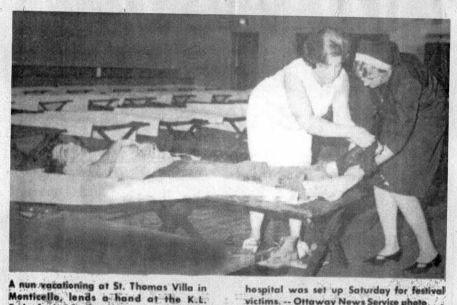

A nun vacationing at St. Thomas Villa in Monticello, lends a hand at the K.L. Rutherford School where an emergency hospital was set up Saturday for festival victims. -- Ottaway News Service photo.

evening, a reasonable amount of order had been established here.

Dr. Alan Fried came down from his medical practice in Livingston Manor, 20 miles away, to assist at the Rutherford School. He remembers how close the cots were and was particularly "impressed that each patient came with a friend or two. None came alone."[28] Monticello Doctors Kornbluh and Lipson helped out, along with others whose names are lost to time. Monticello physician Herman Goldfarb, spent all day Saturday and into Sunday morning treating patients at the Monticello Hospital emergency room. Nurses Anna Benson, Patti Van Etten and Hildur Hindley of Monticello also pitched in at the Rutherford School for long periods.

Benson remembers assessing a six-month-old girl with severe sunburn and dehydration. Local pediatrician Dr. Gustave Gavis directed her to rush the infant and the child's mother to the Monticello Hospital by car, as there were no ambulances available.

As Ann drove the mother and daughter to the hospital in her car, she commented to the mother, "The baby should be with her grandmother," to which the mother replied, "No, she shouldn't."

Eighteen-year-old Monticello native Howard Perlman helped out with supplies at the hastily set-up infirmary, but took the opportunity to go to the festival site in a station wagon to pick up a fair-goer with a badly injured leg and bring him back to the Rutherford School.

Another Monticello teen, Harvey Lashinsky, learned through the town's motorcycle club that couriers were needed. He fired up his dirt bike and volunteered. "I went back and forth from the Rutherford School four or five times to deliver medical supplies to the triage tent at the festival," he said.[29]

Injuries ranged from heat prostration to cuts and bruises to drug reactions. One teenager was found recuperating there Sunday morning; the roast beef sandwich he was eating was the first food he'd had since Thursday. He had fainted at the festival.

Dr. Schiff coordinated the effort there, along with Community General Hospital Board President Gordon Winarick and executives Mischa Leshner and A. F. Cacchillo. Monticello school board president Dr. Russel Pantel and school superintendent Charles Rudiger saw to it that things ran smoothly at the school. Twenty nuns vacationing at St. Thomas Villa in Monticello showed up to lend a hand. They were members of the Sisters of St. Joseph, an order founded in 1650 to promote universal fellowship and social justice. One addled patient woke up, saw the sisters, and reported afterward, "I thought I was dead and in heaven."[30]

A number of local doctors saw patients in their offices during the festival. Most prominent of these was Dr. Sol Dombeck, who operated his practice out of his home, which was located on Route 17B just past the White Lake traffic light and less than 3 miles from the Hurd Road turn-off to the festival grounds. As this stretch of road was impassible except by foot or motorcycle because of the traffic jam, tens of thousands of young people trekked past his door.

Among the many Dombeck cared for was Richard J. Malloy, a fair-goer from Schenectady, New York. Sixteen years later, Malloy got around to sending the doctor a thank-you note and payment for his services. "At that time you treated a badly cut foot (mine) and also fed a very hungry person (me)," Malloy wrote. " . . . I never forgot your help." He included a check for $25.[31]

Dr. Gustave Gavis, the Bethel Town Health Director, traveled between the triage center, the festival site, and local hospitals. He was impressed by the dedication and spontaneous coordination of those working on the medical effort. "This was a voluntary emergency thing. . . . Whatever was done, we didn't have a dictator. People would say, 'You need something? I'll do it. You want to open the school? We'll open the school.' People worked together."[32]

Volunteers at the Monticello Jewish Center assembled 10,000 sandwiches, which were airlifted in, along with 10,000 more provided by the Concord Hotel.

The New York Times

WITH A LITTLE HELP FROM HER FRIENDS: Girl with an injured foot getting a lift at Woodstock fair yesterday.

Soup stations were set up in Monticello's De Hoyos Memorial park to feed the many who had not reached the site or were in retreat from it. Local stores donated milk, bread, and meat.

After helping out at the Rutherford School on Saturday, Helen Reno went to the St. Peter's School, also in Monticello, which had opened its doors to the many who had congregated in town who had no food or shelter. Red Cross volunteers helped out with cots;

church members who taught Culinary Arts at Sullivan County Community College help to prepare donated food. According to Monsignor Edward Straub, assistant pastor at St. Peter's in Monticello at the time, about 400 people were helped over the three days.

A group that included various clergy associations of Sullivan County had agreed with Woodstock Ventures to provide counselors at the festival's "rap tent" on the festival grounds. Msgr. Straub manned the rap tent from noon to 8:00 p.m. on Friday. Volunteers there provided counseling for non-drug problems. Father Peter Malet, then assistant pastor of St. Peter's in Liberty, was flown into the festival site by helicopter to perform Mass on Saturday at 5:00 p.m. at the festival's Meditation Gardens.

With help coming from a variety of directions, the medical situation at festival itself began to stabilize. A mimeograph flyer that Hog Farm members distributed around 8:00 p.m. Saturday summed up the situation and gave advice. It reported "crowded but improving medical facilities." It exhorted the young people not to be "passive consumers of music. . . . Life could get hard . . . pull together in the spirit of the Catskill mountain guerilla, and share — everything will be cool." It went on:

> There are three medical stations. Minor stuff (cuts and bruises) can be taken care of at the South Station in the Hog Farm, or at the health trailer at the main intersection (behind the stage). A plane load of doctors has been airlifted from New York City. Medical supplies have been flown in and patients are being flown out every fifteen minutes. Serious injuries will be treated at the large red and white tent behind the information booth located at the west corner of the stage area. Drug freakouts will be tended by Hog Farm people (red armbands). Any trained medical personnel should report to the above medical centers. //

Many freakouts. Do not take acid from strangers, and understand that taking strong dope may be a drag when your help is needed. // Do not run naked in the hot sun for any period of time (do it in the shade). You're risking water loss and severe blisters. // Cuts on bare feet getting quickly infected if not treated. // People using chronic medications should report to medical centers for refills, but don't wait.[33]

More tetanus toxoid was flown in. The stream of patients with cut feet kept coming. Thorough cleansing of wounds was a time-consuming process for the nurses, volunteers and doctors, but it saved many festival-goers from serious infection. If the wound was deep, a plastic bag was attached around the foot after the patient was treated. Otherwise, gauze and an Ace bandage sufficed.

Somewhere along the line, Thomas Kracht, an ambulance attendant with Sullivan County Ambulance fell down in utter exhaustion after 48 hours without rest. He slept two hours and went back on duty.

The Music

Friday was intended for folkies, starting with the hypnotic guitar rhythms of Richie Havens. Tim Hardin, Arlo Guthrie, and The Incredible String Band were also on the bill. Joan Baez sang about the martyred union organizer Joe Hill, who had been hanged around the time the grandparents of the Woodstock generation were themselves teenagers.

Saturday was the day for rock and roll. The Grateful Dead, Santana, and Janis Joplin performed before the appreciative crowds. The Who came on and played late into the night.

Sunday saw Jefferson Airplane, Joe Cocker, Johnny Winter, and The Band. Again, the music stretched on all night. Jimi Hendrix didn't come on until 9:00 a.m. Monday morning.

Dr. Abruzzi went into Monticello on Saturday and asked to take a shower at the home of a local pharmacist. Overcome by fatigue, he slept for twenty minutes. He found time for two more hours of sleep on Sunday.

Abbie Hoffman marveled later about the spontaneous eruption of a sense of community. "The way people responded, how they volunteered, how they became so professional at this so quickly, it was absolutely wonderful, wonderful."[34]

By Sunday, the danger of an immediate crisis had passed. Helicopters were flying out fewer patients—the Army helicopters took out 39 patients Sunday, compared to 58 on Saturday evening. Some festival goers were headed for home, particularly after additional heavy rain and storms on Sunday afternoon.

The most severe of the thunderstorms caught the folks in the hospital tent unaware and threatened to overturn it. Nurses held down the poles and scrambled to keep bandages and other supplies from getting wet.

The music continued before a diminishing crowd through Sunday night. The promoters worried about rioting or other violence if the music stopped. They encouraged performers to play extended sets, said operations director Mel Lawrence, "because we had to keep the crowd cool."[35] Each act pushed the schedule back farther. The music went on all night and was still blasting when the sun came up.

Jimi Hendrix, the headliner, insisted on appearing last. He took the stage not at midnight on Sunday, as planned, but around 9:00 a.m. Monday morning. By that time the crowd had dwindled to about 60,000 spectators.

As Hendrix played his extended and distorted version of the national anthem, some fans had heard enough. "I remember trying to fall asleep during the 'Star-Spangled Banner,'" one fair-goer said. "I just wished he would stop."[36]

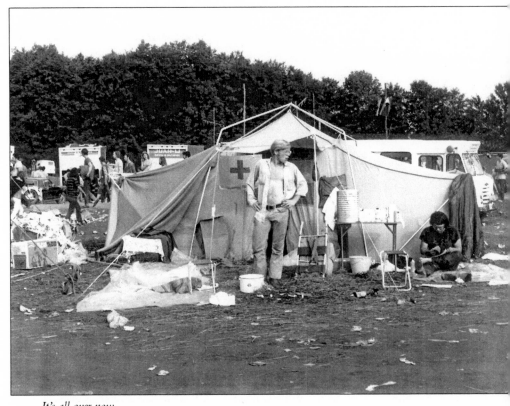

It's all over now

4

~~~~~~~~~~~~~~~

A Little Heaven

R. ABRUZZI stayed on with a skeleton crew for another few days to care for the stragglers as dazed young people hunted for lost cars and lost friends. Dr. Boor returned to treat some of the Hog Farmers, who were involved in the arduous cleanup and had developed respiratory ailments. But for all intents and purposes, Woodstock ended on Monday.

Given the chaotic conditions that availed through most of the festival, the records that Dr. Abruzzi compiled were remarkably precise. Whether he was able to maintain a running log of the activities of his staff and the hundreds of volunteers during the three days, or whether his figures represent estimates transformed into statistics for the bureaucrats in Albany, is impossible to determine.

Some medical people remember names and symptoms being recorded as patients entered the makeshift facilities, but no detailed prehospital care reports were written up.

Mischa Leshner, the Community General Hospital official who helped set up the Rutherford School triage center, noted, "I think we wrote down the names of people, if they told us. . . . But I don't think we made out any ER sheets." In part this was a strategy on the part of hospital officials to avoid having to report patients with drug overdoses to the police by name. According to Leshner, records were listed under headings like "Male X," "Female Y."[1]

Abruzzi's figures represent the best summary available of the weekend's medical toll. Beyond the precise figures, Abruzzi estimated a total of 3,000 people were treated at the site.

Injuries to feet were the most common ailment. Abruzzi lists 938 lacerations in his official report, along with 135 punctures and 346 other foot injuries.

Abruzzi and his staff treated people at the festival from 40 states, ranging in age from newborn to elderly. He noted a number of surprises: The 23 epileptic seizures treated were more than would have been expected, given the crowd size. So were the 176 cases of asthma requiring therapy. But only nine patients presented with venereal disease, fewer than what Abruzzi would have expected to see.

The fact that only 86 patients were diagnosed with gastroenteritis, was "incredible" under the conditions, he reported. The mud, inadequate toilet facilities, and crowded environment would have argued for more stomach upsets.[2]

Wouldn't Have Missed It

Ivan "Hy" Zimmerman was director of special activities at Homowack Lodge, a popular resort in Spring Glen, about thirty miles from Bethel. Homowack was one of many resorts in the area that contributed needed supplies in the emergency. Zimmerman traveled to the festival with food supplies donated by the resort and took along his own medical equipment. A licensed practical nurse, he became aware of the need for medical people and signed on for the duration. He was assigned to the pink hospital tent.

Zimmerman administered something like 500 tetanus shots during his stint at the festival. The storm that came on Sunday "would have blown our hospital tent away if not for the volunteers who came in from the festival to hold down the poles."

He stayed on through Monday. "I wouldn't have missed it for the world."[3]

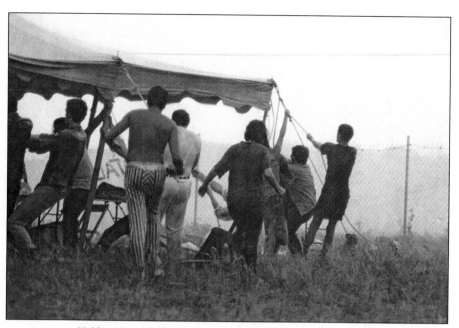
Holding down the hospital tent in the storm

In spite of surviving three days marked by violent storms, often with inadequate shelter and exposed to heat that ranged up to 95 degrees, only 30 fair-goers came to the medical facilities because of headache, 57 for "heat exhaustion," 64 for exposure to cold, and 87 for "exhaustion and fatigue."

Other ailments were about what would have been expected from a crowd of that size. Two people experienced ruptured appendixes. There were five miscarriages, referred to in medical jargon as incomplete abortions. Three cases of noncommunicable hepatitis. Twelve cases of food poisoning. The fact that cases of food-borne illness were limited was attributed by some observers to the fact that what food was available was consumed so quickly that there was little chance of spoilage.

One of the problems that the nurses dealt with was that of young mothers who had left their nursing babies home to attend the fair. Pollets remembered applying hot compresses to swollen breasts and

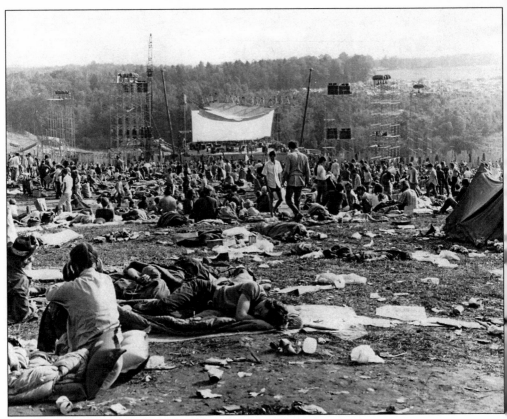

Monday morning

instructing the young mothers about how to express their milk. "I said, 'Go home, go home and feed your baby.' That bothered me that they left their babies home with their grandmas."[4]

Quite a few injuries were the result of falls from cars and motorcycles. "The kids were riding on bumpers, roofs, anywhere," said Sheriff Louis Ratner.[5] Broken toes and fingers were treated, along with stomach sickness, flu, infections, poison ivy, and heat prostration.

Monticello physician Dr. Lester Lipson reported three cases of ulcers of the eyes because people had left their contacts in for as much as three days. One of these had to be sent to a hospital in Newburgh.

According to Abruzzi's final report, 250 patients were evacuated by helicopters to hospitals.

Not all patients were satisfied with their treatment. A girl came to the first aid facilities with a broken toe. Doctors there gave her some Darvon and told her they could do nothing else. Faced with nine-mile walk to her car, she succumbed to tears.

Another girl could not find her car after traipsing up and down the roads for five mile and was also unable to locate her sister. Overwhelmed, she had to lie down in the medical tent. But after a rest and a glass of water, she ventured out to resume her search.

A chubby boy with glasses couldn't find anywhere to sleep. A doctor reported him immature and frightened. Unable to find relief at the first aid center, he simply set out walking.

A nurse remembered tending to one girl's injured foot. "I never saw such feet in my life." The girl had calluses on her feet "like a shoe." When the nurse warned her that she would never be able to fit her feet into "a pair of decent ladies' shoes," the girl said she didn't care. The doctor fixed her up, and lacking both socks and shoes, "Away she went."[6]

Doctor C.B. Esselstyn, who was heading the State's Bureau of Emergency Medical Services stated in his evaluation, "I felt the medical coverage was well organized under the direction of Dr. William Abruzzi." He noted at least temporary shortages of Valium, dilantin, tetanus toxoid, and sanitary napkins.

But he concluded, "In spite of the emergency which was created by the overwhelming, unexpected number, I believe the health problems were handled expeditiously. The cooperative spirit and orderly conduct of this mass of humanity facilitated the overworked skeleton medical team."[7]

The Board of Trustees of Community General Hospital later calculated that they handed over $3,423.89 worth of medical supplies and drugs and sent Woodstock Ventures a bill.

"The response of the nurses, doctors, medical records librarians, etc. from both Divisions, was magnificent," their report noted. "The whole matter was handled extremely well and is a credit to the Hospital. In fact, the Hospital was the only agency that planned for the Festival, setting up and using a variety of its disaster plan."

The board went on to note that "plans should be formulated, based on this experience, for emergences and disasters of every nature."[8]

The Monticello School Board also noted the contributions of their people, including "Dr. Pantel, Mrs. Mitchell, Mrs. Field, Dr. Rudiger, Mr. Pollack and others on the school staff." On Sunday night they had sent out a school bus to transport walkers along Route 17B to the Short Line bus terminal.[9]

Sullivan County Ambulance Service owner Thomas McFarlin noted that his people had handled more than 300 calls, taking patients from the grounds to the tent hospital, or from there to the helicopter landing zone. They also delivered patients to areas hospitals and transported others from the Rutherford School triage center to hospitals.

McFarlin's ambulances sustained $2,800 in damages from burned-out transmissions and cut tires. Drivers had to be careful driving, watching out for people lying under blankets or in sleeping bags. McFarlin noted that at no time was any ambulance stuck in the mud for more than five minutes – there were always plenty of volunteers ready to push it out.

The Drug Toll

The Woodstock Festival has a reputation as an orgy of drugs plagued by innumerable "freakouts" and overdoses. Were there a lot of bad trips? Abruzzi, who was nonjudgmental about recreational drug use, recorded a total of 797 bad trips that needed some supportive care. But of those, only 72 were seen by a doctor and 28 were treated with

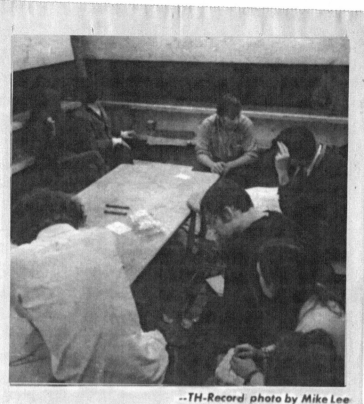

--TH-Record photo by Mike Lee

The inside of one of the medical centers for kids who are on bad trips from .... drugs.

medication. The vast majority responded to supportive therapy only.

One observer pointed out that the impression of a mass freakout was not surprising. For most people, seeing twenty people freak out means "you've seen twenty times more freakouts than you've ever seen in your life, and that seems like a lot."[10]

Tom Law, one of the Hog Farmers, concluded, "There were very few bad drugs."[11] Indeed, no inadvertent poisoning or prolonged, drug-induced psychosis was reported.

To put Woodstock in perspective, it's interesting to look at other outdoor rock festivals. In August 1970, the Powder Ridge Festival was scheduled to take place near Middlefield, Connecticut. Dr.

Abruzzi, whose experience would gain him the moniker "Rock Doc," was again in charge of the medical treatment. The crowd was estimated at between 20,000 and 35,000, less than a tenth of the mass of folks at Woodstock. There, medical personnel treated 985 bad trips, almost 200 more than at Woodstock.

Admittedly, Powder Ridge was a bit of a bummer to begin with since none of the scheduled band played after local officials filed an injunction against the festival as a public nuisance. But the much higher incidence of bad drug reactions is striking and indicates that Woodstock could have been much worse.

Another interesting comparison is with the Altamont Speedway Free Festival held outside San Francisco on December 6, 1969. The event was built around an appearance by the Rolling Stones and included Jefferson Airplane, Santana and other groups that had played at Woodstock a few months earlier. The concert was notorious for the murder of 18-year-old Meredith Hunter by Hell's Angels members hired to furnish security. The one-day event was also marred by three accidental deaths and numerous injuries from fights. The lack of anything resembling a freakout tent or compassionate care for drug users meant the bad trip problem at Altamont was also more serious than at Woodstock.

Birth

Were babies born at Woodstock? Numerous reports said there were. Abbie Hoffman asserted there were "maybe three or four births."[12] Carol Green, who worked as a cook for the festival, also said, "There were three or four births."[13]

Doctor Esselstyn, the state EMS director, wrote in a report that "two girls went into labor," but did not elaborate.[14]

A reporter for the local Times Herald-Record sent his editor a flash: *There apparently is a baby being delivered in the medical hospital at the festival site. Delivery right now.* That paper also mentioned a "report a couple of girls have given birth on festival site."[15]

On Monday, the newspaper reported that one birth occurred in a car going "either in or out" and another in a local hospital "after the mother was evacuated." A third birth was "to take place here after doctors decided not to move the mother. The mother was in a tent within earshot of Sunday's music show."[16]

Dr. Jack Maidman was a New York obstetrician who had seen the Monterey Pop festival film and was determined to take in the spectacle at Woodstock. While at the festival, he checked in at the medical tent and told the staff there that he was willing to help out if needed. They said they would page him over the festival loudspeakers.

No too long afterward, there was an announcement for him to come to the medical tent "with full suture kit" because a woman was about to give birth. The call proved to be a false alarm, but it and other stage announcements planted images of an imminent birth in thousands of brains.

Announcement From the Stage

Fibber McGee, please come immediately to back stage right. I understand your wife is having a baby. Congratulations!

All these casual reports and notions solidified into a persistent myth that one or more babies were born on the festival grounds.

But Record editor Al Romm noted, "There were supposedly a handful of births that took place. We couldn't find proof of it in the aftermath. It was just a rumor."[17]

He noted that ABC network researchers tried to track down the authenticity of the rumor for either the tenth or fifteenth anniversary of Woodstock, hoping to talk to the kid born there. But local hospitals could provide no evidence to confirm the story.

Elliot Tiber, who helped run his parents' motel El Monaco in nearby White Lake includes in a book about the era a graphic account of a would-be festival goer giving birth in one of his rooms. "A tiny Woodstock baby girl was born into my arms."[18] The child and mother were transported from the motel by helicopter, Tiber reports. Years later, Tiber was still trying to locate the baby.

A recollection from a volunteer at the festival adds another wrinkle to the story. Gladys Devaney, a member of the Town of Liberty Volunteer Ambulance Corps, remembers a woman in labor in the medical tent. As she was being moved by stretcher to an ambulance, the birth became imminent. Devaney, trained in first aid, attempted to guide the baby as it emerged, but it "slipped out of my hands onto the stretcher mattress. It wasn't hurt and was breathing and looked good."

The baby and mother were immediately whisked away and Devaney remembers nothing more about the incident, not even the infant's gender.

In spite of all the reports, myths, and conflicting accounts, it's still an open question whether any baby emerged from the womb on the grounds of the great Aquarian Festival. Doctors who served in Sullivan County's only obstetrics practice at the time reported that they knew of no out-of-hospital births or obstetrical emergencies during the weekend.

Both Dr. Abruzzi and the New York Times reported two births. One took place in a car that was stuck in traffic near to the festival. The other involved a woman who went into labor at the festival and was airlifted to a hospital. Because of privacy laws, hospital records are not available to shed light on the question.

Joel Makower, who compiled an oral history of the Woodstock festival, has a theory about why no one has ever come forward to make the claim.

"The mother is now a respectable citizen, a schoolteacher, let's say, in a small community in upstate New York," he said, "and does not want the world to know she gave birth in an alfalfa field in Sullivan County. This mother, for the same reason she doesn't want to tell the world, hasn't even told her child."[19]

Good Vibes

"There was no disaster, no holocaust, catastrophe, riot, havoc, nightmare, or any major confrontation." That was the verdict of Gerald Lieber, of the Department of Health, in a report summarizing the Woodstock Festival.

"All the necessary ingredients were there," he went on, "an unexpectedly large number of spectators, two heavy rainstorms . . .

Amazed and Changed

One volunteer was the 15-year-old high school freshman Michael Baxter, who had purchased a ticket for Sunday's concert, but whose parents wouldn't let him go. When the call went out for first-aid volunteers, Baxter's mother Ruth answered the call.

Baxter had a Red Cross basic first aid card himself and was a junior member of the Mountaindale Fire Department First Aid Squad, twenty miles from Bethel. He accompanied his mother into the grounds by helicopter.

"My 'medical' task was mostly washing people's really dirty feet that were cut and scraped," he remembered.

He was scared and intrigued by his first overdose, "a guy lying on a cot, pretty comatose." He soon lost interest in his "first aid gig," and wandered out to explore the surreal scene around him.

What stayed with him was not the bands, the naked people, or the drugs, "but rather the effect Woodstock had on my mother." A conservative country woman with nothing good to say about hippies, she found Woodstock a revelation. Impressed by the people and attitudes she encountered and the lack of violence, "she was truly amazed and changed by what she saw."[23]

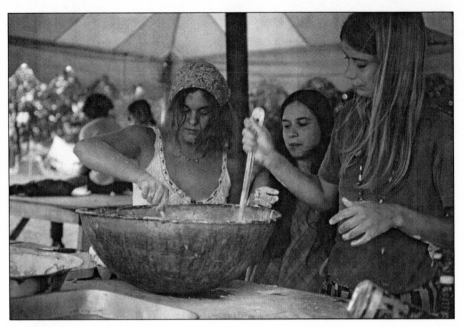

Making the mush

inadequate roads, ... many youngsters having come partially and in some cases totally unprepared ..."[20]

Yet the weekend came off better than anyone could have anticipated, and far better than some feared during the hairy early hours. Lieber concluded that the event suffered "no serious health or sanitary problems at any time during the three-day weekend." The question is, Why?

Lieber suggested that order was maintained "possibly through the use of various drugs and narcotics which may have kept many in a docile mood throughout the festival weekend."[21] This is a remarkable statement. A few years after Woodstock, the administration of Governor Nelson Rockefeller, for whom Lieber worked, enacted the so-called "Rockefeller drug laws," which made the possession of four ounces of any "narcotic," including marijuana, punishable by a long, mandatory prison sentence. Lieber was asserting that those same drugs had contributed to maintaining public order in a perilous situation.

Dr. Abruzzi did not subscribe to the notion that everyone was too stoned to cause trouble. Rather, he said, an atmosphere of "love, tolerance, and forbearance" prevailed. "Hospitals and staff worked overtime. Ambulance drivers, attendants, and volunteers staggered through miles of mud laden with stretchers bearing their fellow human beings in need."

Those who had food and drink shared it. Those who had to wait two hours to use a pay phone or stand in line to visit a Port-a-Potty did not complain.

"The weekend could have been a tragedy of mammoth proportions," Abruzzi said later. "Rather than medical preparations, I think it was good fortune that saved us."[22]

Any group of people, even one as impromptu and amorphous as the hordes who descended on Bethel that weekend, takes on a character. A mood, an expectation, unspoken norms of behavior suffuse the crowd and rule more surely than any law imposed by the larger society. Call it a vibe.

Observers of all kinds – participants, doctors, promoters, police officers, skeptical local residents – agree that the vibe at Woodstock was polite, good humored, mellow. And it was that mood, more than anything, that averted the disaster that might have been.

The hero of Woodstock, by many accounts, was Hog Farm leader Wavy Gravy. More than any other individual, he helped generate the spirit that permeated the festival. He was far more in tune with

Breakfast in Bed

Many fair-goers, accustomed to pizza and hot dogs, found Sunday's breakfast a bit unusual. The Hog Farmers cooked rolled oats or bulgur wheat into a mush. They added peanuts, creating a goulash consistency. Vegetables from neighboring farms, when available, were stir-fried and heaped on the side, everything dished up on a paper plate.

what was happening than many of the musicians, who remained insulated inside their bubbles of celebrity.

To begin with, Wavy provided expert guidance for those trippers on the edge of insanity. It's not difficult to imagine the hundreds of seriously out-of-control LSD-using individuals setting off hysteria or panic in the large crowd. Instead, these patients were treated with patience, kindness, understanding, and human contact. Their mania did not become contagious.

Wavy also provided an injection of humor into the body politic of the festival. Having been a professional comedian on the club circuit – Lenny Bruce was once his manager – he knew how to get his own funny view of the world across to the masses. As an informal master of ceremonies, he helped everyone to look on the trying conditions as a joke rather than a catastrophe.

By the third day food was running low. "What we have in mind," Wavy announced on Sunday morning, "is breakfast in bed for four hundred thousand. It's going to be good food and we're going to get it to you."[24]

But the success of Woodstock could not be attributed to one man. The real hero of the festival was the crowd itself, the Woodstock Generation. They made up their minds to behave decently, not to be provoked by weather or abominable conditions or each other. In their addled way, they took responsibility. They were the performers more than any musicians, and they made a good show of it. As a result, instead of infectious disease, there was infectious good will.

"My idea of Woodstock is that we had a chance to either be in a disaster area or uplevel the whole game," said Wavy's wife Jahanara. "And we chose to uplevel the whole game. . . . There was a transformation of human beings that took place that was cosmic or spiritual or whatever word one would use for a higher level of interacting with people."[25]

Members of the counterculture were not the only ones who

were impressed by the spirit that had emerged during the three days. Ben Filipino, a land owner in Bethel, called the event "the seventh wonder of the world." Monticello police chief Lou Yank said festival goers were "the most courteous, considerate group of kids."[26] *CBS Evening News* commentator John Lawrence noted that "in an emergency at least, people of all ages are capable of real compassion."[27]

Woodstock was designed to make bucks, Wavy Gravy noted. "Then the universe took over and did a little dance." [28]

Speaking of the difficult conditions at the festival, Dr. Abruzzi noted that "from this climate of deprivation, crowding and difficulty can come a feeling of love, tolerance, and forbearance such as we should all envy."

He went on to point out what was perhaps the most noteworthy fact connected to the medical aspect of the gathering. In spite of the massive crowd, in spite of the rain, the mud, the shortages, and the widespread drug use, at no time did anyone on the medical team see or treat "any incident, which involved the causing of personal or physical injury from one human being to another. Not a knife wound was sewed, not a punch wound was treated."

Peace and love really did prevail. Abruzzi added, "Christ would have smiled."[29]

Appendix

1. William Abruzzi, M.D., "A White Lake Happening," report to New York State Department of Health, September 2, 1969.

2. Gerald Lieber, P.E., Senior Sanitary Engineer, Monticello Subdistrict; report to New York State Department of Health, September 8, 1969.

3. C.B. Esselstyn, M.D., Director of Emergency Medical Services, New York State Department of Health; reports to New York State Department of Health, August 19, 1969.

4. C.B. Esselstyn, M.D., Director of Emergency Medical Services, New York State Department of Health; reports to New York State Department of Health, September 8, 1969.

5. Abbie Hoffman, "Survival Sheet."

6. Dr. Dombeck letter

7. New York State Department of Health, "Permit to Operate a Temporary Residence."

8. Wesley A. Pomeroy, Security Consultant. Woodstock Ventures, Inc. Page 3 of Security Plan, "Aquarian Festival" Bethel, New York, August 15, 16 & 17, 1969.

9. Sullivan County Ambulance Service.

10. Mobilemedic 51-93 (2008 American Emergency Vehicles, Type II).

11. The Musuem at Bethel Woods Center for the Arts.

12. Max Yasgur's statement about the 1969 Woodstock Music Festival.

1. William Abruzzi, M.D., "A White Lake Happening," report to New York State Department of Health, September 2, 1969.

"A White Lake Happening"

It starts out like a simple tale. I was asked to do something I've done several times before. I was asked to set up a health facility, along emergency room, or field hospital lines, to take care of the medical needs of 50,000 plus people at a folk-rock festival to be held in Sullivan County, New York, August 1969. This didn't seem like a terribly difficult challenge. To recruit 18 doctors (two for each 8 hour shifts for 72 hours) and similarly assign 36 nurses, four for each shift, and 27 medical assistants, three for each shift; and to equip and outfit and make ready for operation, one or two medical trailers with minor surgical equipment, etc; to coordinate ambulance evacuation facilities; to arrange with local hospitals for the overflow; to set up two or three hospital tent facilities in order to take care of resting patients, patients to be evacuated, and emergencies that could not easily be removed; all of this seemed rather routine. After all, it shouldn't be too different from setting up a field hospital facility in the Mississippi delta, or arranging for the medical care of 40,000 to 50,000 people on one of the southern civil rights marches. Inspection of hospital facilities (already overworked with summer vacation crowds and sufficiently small so as to be without intensive care units or housestaffs) aerial and ground inspection of road accessibility, and on-site evaluation of a rolling farmland, essentially vulnerable to wind, rain and mud, led one to begin to have second thoughts. A helicopter appraisal of the situation on Friday, the first day of the festival, revealed a crowd approaching which was frightening in its aspects. The turn-off lanes on Route 17 were clogged from Monticello to the Thruway. The Thruway turn-off lanes on to Route 17 were clogged almost

back to the George Washington Bridge. The unbelievable aspects of the
possibility of there being more than 200,000 people converging on the
Exposition site began to convey medical responsibility apprehensions to me.
A consultation with the executive officers of the Exposition gave me complete
freedom to engage any help necessary, incorporate any procedures or steps
required, and overall, to add to the medical facility whatever might be
necessary in order to take care of the larger number of young people. At
this point I had begun to think about the people who had put together the
festival. What sort of people were they? Admittedly, they were young men
interested in making money. Each of them, had in his own way, already proven
his ability to do so. On the otherhand, there were some aspects of this
festival which transcended money-making. For example, if indeed, the only
or primary motivation of the festival was financial, then why had more than
a hundred people from the New Mexico "Hog Farm" been flown at Exposition
expense to New York in order to aid in the preparation for the event and care
of the anticipated number of "freakouts" - the young people whose trip on
drugs would not necessarily be an easy or good one. In addition, why the
extras which gave the entire affair more artistic and sensory value? Why the
great stone swing? Why the artistically constructed rabbit hutch and chicken
runs? Why the huge and imaginative sandbox and playpen? Certainly, this was
not the mark of people only concerned with making money. After all, the people
who bought the tickets would have no way of knowing that these extras were available
to them when they purchased them. Their attitude concerning the expansion of
the medical facility, and that no stone should be unturned to give complete
and adequate health care to everyone present, further

New York State Department of Health
Albany Regional Office
Taxation and Finance Bldg. (#9)
Room 412

2

bolsters the conclusion that there was much more involved here than finances.

From one medical trailer and two hospital tents, the facilities were able to be developed. Workmen appeared magically, new wall hospital tents were constructed, floors were installed, lighting was instituted, phones were strung, doctors and nurses were recruited from nearby and far-off places. Repeated trips by helicopter resulted in the acquisition of medical and surgical supplies sufficient to care for many additional hundreds of thousands. Psychiatrists were flown in from New York to run special psychiatric and "trip" clinics. All in all, a health facility sufficient to care for 1/3 to 1/2 million people began to take shape. Those medical personnel, who had already been assigned, worked around the clock, and relief groups began to appear. The Medical Committee for Human Rights donated personnel and equipment, and a Middletown State Hospital made available to us supplies which were urgently needed.

But then, the problems began to compound themselves. With each additional 100,000 young people who appeared on the scene, the problem didn't simply become that of increasing the medical facility to care for 100,000 more people. Instead, the roads became more clogged; the food situation became more acute; the water replacement problems became more difficult; the sanitation crews became more and more overburdened; the telephone and toilet facility lines became longer; the bathing facilities became more difficult; all in all the problems didn't just add to each other, they seemed to multiply and to cause concurrent problems in other areas. And then the heavens intervened! Three separate and distinct violent storms racked the area during the festival. The winds

New York State Department of Health
Albany Regional Office
Taxation and Finance Bldg. (#9)
Room 412
State Office Building Campus

blew to a point where hospital tents had to be forcibly held down by
hundreds of volunteers. The rains came until the pasture land was nothing
but a morass of mud; and the problems grew apace. The water problem became
even more difficult due to the mud and rain. The shelter problems became
almost impossible due to the wind and rain; the medical and health problems
abounded as all were exposed to the elements and as their dry clothing
disappeared, their shelter became useless, and cleanliness became next to
impossible. There was a corollary to this which no one could have anticipated
and which caused more difficulty than anything else. As a result of the
tremendous depth of the muck and mud which resulted from the downpours, most
shoes and sandals were lost. As a result, the majority of the boys and girls
were barefoot by the end of the second day. Similiarly, as a result, our
foot problems medically multiplied. Almost every other case which appeared
for first aid was a case of foot injury or foot laceration and/or puncture
wound. Instead of treating the anticipated or projected estimate of a
couple of hundred foot cases, we were treating well over two thousand cases.
This, in turn, was not only a burden on medical personnel and equipment, but
more than anything else caused us to be continually and repeatedly short of
tetanus toxoid. As a result, the emergency calls for replenishing supplies
of tetanus toxoid went out Sunday and Monday until supplies were flown to
us from as far away as Rockland County, and almost every available vial of
tetanus toxoid in Sullivan County was utilized for our purposes.

A situation of potential medical emergency was declared and as a result
civil defense and the U. S. Army were invaluable to us over the last 24 to 48
hours of the festival. A civil defense facility was set up near Monticello

New York State Department of Health
Albany Regional Office
Taxation and Finance Bldg. (#9)
Room 412

126

in a high school, which served as a clearing house and field hospital unit.
Army helicopters, large and able to evacuate 4 to 6 people at a time, similar
to those used in Vietnam, were pressed into service. Stewart Field was able
to be used for landing the patients who needed large hospital facility care
and could then be evacuated to St. Luke's Hospital, Newburgh, New York.
Ambulance crews in every surrounding township were put on the alert and made
available to us in emergencies during that critical time. Physicians, first
aid facilities, and hospital facilities for miles around were alerted and
responsive to the emergent needs of the situation.

In the meantime, what was happening on the site? What were we doing
about the medical care of the nearly half a million people? How were we
getting to the people who needed medical attention? How were we getting them to
a facility which could care for them? For example, one medical facility on
the Exposition site was almost three miles from another. How could a patient
who needed care at one or the other be transported thereto? An ambulance
could not manage the muddy farm wagon roads from one place to another in the
middle of a storm. Many of us learned the kind of physical condition we were
in by having to transport a patient on a stretcher two or three miles. The
patients who were in need of psychiatric or personal attention as a result of
drug overdose, had to be transported from the first area to an area near the
hog farm. The patients at the hog farm who needed possible evacuation for medical
problems needed to be transported to the "pink and white" hospital tent. These
were logistic and mechanical problems which awaited us. Because everyone
participated, because everyone cooperated, because everyone cared, the entire
operation was able to be successful. On Saturday afternoon, repeated

helicopter trips by State Police and others brought to us a sobering statistic. It was estimated at that time that there were over 1/3 of a million people at the exposition site. It was further estimated (and this was by far the more frightening statistic) that there were as many as possibly still a million people on the way. It was at this point that rather frantic appeals, some of them from me, and some of them from the festival officials, some from State officials, went out to the news media to people who had not yet arrived to turn back before they helped to compound the tremendous problem of too many people in one spot. I think it was then that we all realized for the first time the propensity for having the greatest medical tragedy of our times. Certainly, the influx of another million people or any significant proportion thereof, would have created a medical situation which no number of doctors, or nurses, no amount of medical and surgical supplies could have conceivably compensated for. In addition, the problem of evacuating that number after the Exposition was over, would have been close to insurmountable, and would have resulted in a health facility having to remain for another week or two after the Exposition ended. How effective were our appeals to turn back radioed to those who had not yet arrived, we will never know. Suffice it to say that the number of people collected apparently never exceeded the figure given on Sunday which was 480,000.

What kind of medical experience did we have in terms of statistics? We treated young people from well over 40 states. We treated people in age from newborn, 2, 3, and 4 week old infants up to the very elderly and aged. It has been intimated above that the largest category of treated cases was in the area of foot problems. There were 938 lacerations of the feet. There were 346 other injuries to the foot. There were 135 puncture wounds

New York State Department of Health
Albany Regional Office

of the feet. There were almost 250 patients evacuated by helicopters to various hospital facilities one of which was simply a clearing house and evacuation hospital type facility. These ranged from fractures, to epilepsy, threatened and incomplete abortion, appendicitis, etc. From previous experience of the health care of 50,000 to 100,000 people it was easy to project the number of diabetics that would be in coma or in shock, the cardiac problems that would be treated, the number of cases of epilepsy that might be seen, the number of emotional problems that might occur, the number of cases of infectious, gastrointestinal and upper respiratory disease that might prove a problem, etc. There were a few more surprises which we must add to our knowledgeability about "crowd" medicine in the future: For example, 23 epileptic seizures seemed like more than we had a right to expect for that number of people for three days. 176 cases of asthma requiring therapy in that period of time, more than one might expect? Isn't nine cases of venereal disease a smaller number than one might expect? And isn't it incredible that only 86 cases of gastroenteritis were among 480,000 young people living under conditions that were not altogether perfect and desirable as regards water, food, and sanitation? Doesn't that require some revision in our conceptual images regarding the causation of gastrointestinal diseases and the relation- ship of crowds and sanitation to that causation? Is this terrible "drug scene" of which we hear so much exemplified by the fact that 480,000 kids living together for 3 to 7 days created a total of 797 cases of "trips" that needed some kind of supportive care? Should we think it significant that of those 797, only 72 received any medical attention what-so-ever, and of those 72 only 28 required medication. In other words, 769 so-called overdoses were treated simply with TLC, with supportive therapy, with understanding, with the ego support and

New York State Department of Health
Albany Regional Office
Taxation and F

reward that came from those who understood and cared.

On the other hand, in a 3 to 7 day period punctuated by violent storms, exposure to wind and rain, heat of 90 95 degrees, overcrowding, poor sanitation, food and water conditions at time, would you think that for example, in a similar number of adults, that one would see more than 30 cases of headache, or have only 57 cases complaining of "heat exhaustion," and only 87 cases complaining of "exhaustion and fatigue", and only 64 cases complaining of being cold or wet? This then was the quality of the young person to which we were exposed.

And this brings us to the major conclusions which can be reached from such a medical experience. The conclusions are not necessarily scientific, not necessarily even medical, these conclusions are perhaps better included in the area of philosophy. We have proved, if nothing else, that it is possible to set up a medical facility which can care for one-half million people for any- where from three to seven days. We have proved it is possible to do so on short notice, with limited facilities, with limited road acess, and with almost no ability to compensate for some of the shortages that would result. We have proved also that it is possible for such people under such conditions to live comfortably and happily together. We have been impressed with the fact that from this climate of deprivation, crowding and difficulty can come a feeling of love, tolerance, and forbearance such as we should all envy.

Not one person eating or drinking could be passed without his offering to you a bite or a drink. Not one person complained about a two-hour wait for telephones. Not one person complained of the delay in reaching sanitation-facilities. Not one person was disturbed by a water shortage which sometimes lasted as long as twenty-four hours. No one complained of the cold, the wet, the heat, the mud, the dirt, or the exposure to foot disabilities. An aging electrician rapidly opened sixteen loaves of bread on his car to distribute them to the passing boys and girls. Farmers from miles around saw to it that their eggs were somehow transported at little or no cost to the crowds which were hungry. Near-by homes were open for bathing, toilet, water, and food facilities. The townspeople collected to provide hospital, evacuation, transportation, and food and water facilities for those who could be evacuated to their areas. Hospitals and hospital staffs worked overtime to take care of the overload period. Ambulance drivers, attendants, and volunteers staggered through miles of mud laden with stretchers bearing their fellow humans in need.

And in closing, I leave you with the medical, political, psychological, and philosophical conclusion of this entire affair. At no time during the entire festival did any of the one hundred fifty odd medical personnel who worked at the site treat any case, or see any incident, which involved the causing of personal or physical injury from one human being to another. Not a knife wound was sewed, not a punch wound was treated. This might very well have been an example of the first time that a large number of people have come together, lived together, suffered together, and given to the rest of us an indication that it can be done in love and peace. There was no fish or wine, but perhaps in that spirit, the bread went further, the water lasted longer. Christ would have smiled.

By Doctor Abruzzi

New York State Department of Health
Albany Regional Office
Taxation and Finance Bldg. (#9)
Room 412

Abdominal pain, undiagnosed	33	Eye injury	7
Abdominal pain, secondary to malignant tumor, previously treated	1	Fatigue	37
		Foreign body, hand	3
		Foreign body, foot	92
Abortion, incomplete and complete	8	Fractures	19
		Gastritis	90
Abortion, threatened	12	Gastroenteritis	86
Abrasions and contusions, more than one place	134	Gonorhea	9
		Headache	80
Abscess, hand	1	Heat exhaustion	57
Allergy	112	Hemophilia	1
Anemia	3	Hemorrhoids	4
Anxiety State	163	Hepatitis	8
Appendicitis	2	Hypoglycemia (related to Diabetes?)	4
Arthritis	9		
Asthma	176	Infection, skin	9
Blisters, foot	172	Infection, unspecific	8
Burns	86	Infection, arm	9
Burns, eye	2	Infection, hand	14
Cardiac problems	2	Infection, mouth	10
Chest pain, undiagnosed	5	Infection, foot	77
Concussion	8	Infection, eye	3
Conjunctivitis	39	Injury, hand	93
Constipation	16	Injury, leg	22
Corneal abrasions	43	Injury, foot	346
Cramps, leg	6	Injury, eye	4
Cystitis	34	Injury, rib cage	3
Dehydration	13	Injury, shoulder	4
DT's	3	Injury, arm	3
Dental problems	71	Injury, head	5
Depression (Primary)	4	Injury, ankle	7
Dermatitis	81	Injury, buttock	2
Diabetes	17	Injury, knee	11
Diarrhea, primary (and only)	13	Injury, multiple	11
Digitalis toxicity	2	Insect bites	19
Dislocation, shoulder	2	Lacerations, misc.	3
Dog bite	9	Lacerations, face	5
Dysmenorrhea	9	Lacerations, knee	5
Edema	3	Lacerations, leg and thigh	37
Electric shock	2	Lacerations, hand	176
Epidydymitis	4	Lacerations, side	2
Epilepsy	23	Lacerations, foot	836
Exhaustion and fatigue	87	Lacerations, head	38
Exposure, cold and wet	64	Lacerations, arm	11
Eye infection	6	Laryngitis	2

```
Malnutrition                           11
Monocleosis Infection                   2
Muscular and ligament sprain            2
Neutiris                                1

O.D.:   Acid            333
        Weed             43
        Speed           172
        Heroin            3
        Methedrine        3

        Mescaline       133
        Ritalin           2
        Misc.            53
                        742            742
```

Note: 72 patients seen by medically
trained personnel--Only 28 of the 72
actually rec'd medication, Other 714
were not. They were treated with T.L.C. supportive
encouragement, etc.

```
Otitis                                 37
P.I.D.                                  7
Pharyngitis                            62
Pneumonia                               7
Puncture wound, foot                  135
Pregnancy, (treatment of)               5
Psychosis
   (after over dose or drug withdrawal)  6

a.  Catatonia      2
b.  Paranoia       4

Racoon bite                             1
Rat bite                               11
Rheumatic Fever                         4
Sprain, wrist                           4
Sprain, ankle                           2
Sprain, Leg                             2
Sunburn                                38
Sun (sttoke)                            9
Syncope                                17
Tendon, lacerations                     3
Tonsillitis                            29
Trachea-Bronchitis                     53
Treatment of prosthesis and stump       5
Ulcer, peptic                          16
U.R.I.                                167
Vaginal bleeding(irregular )            2
Vaginitis                               4
Vertigo                                13
Withdrawal, drug                        7
```

2. Gerald Lieber, P.E., Senior Sanitary Engineer, Monticello Subdistrict; report to New York State Department of Health, September 8, 1969.

STATE OF NEW YORK
DEPARTMENT OF HEALTH

MEMORANDUM

~~RECEIVED~~
SEP 8 1969
ONEONTA DIST.,
N. Y. S. DEPT. OF HEALTH

September 4, 1969

To: Dr. Lipari, Oneonta District Office

From: Mr. Lieber, Monticello Sub-District Office

Subject: Report on Activities during the Woodstock Music and Art Festival

There was no disaster, no holocaust, catastrophe, riot, havoc, nightmare, or any major confrontation. All the necessary ingredients were there, an unexpectedly large number of spectators, two heavy rainstorms which created an overbearing mud problem, inadequate roads, causing serious traffic jams and preventing specific vehicles from performing their necessary functions, many youngsters having come partially and in some cases totally unprepared for a weekend event and the presence of uniformed policemen whose presence alone is often the cause of much agitation among the youth of our day. Yet with all these potential volcanoes bubbling beneath the surface, order was maintained through the kindness generated by the State and Local Law Enforcement Agencies and the local townspeople, through the music performed by the giants of these youngsters' musical world and possibly through the use of various drugs and narcotics which may have kept many in a docile mood throughout the festival weekend.

For a period of three days this group of young boys and girls had the power and forces to do as they pleased. Fortunately for all concerned they behaved much as we would have wished and not at all as most of us would have predicted. They displayed a certain oneness, a unity of purpose, a sense of belonging. Their reason for attending the festival was simply that they wanted to see and hear those top recording stars scheduled to perform throughout the weekend. No one expected that this was to be a gathering of some four hundred thousand youngsters in an area not suited for half that number. But once they became a part of this gathering they displayed a remarkable brotherhood towards one another. Sensing that they could not all partake of the festival music, the area in front of the stage and within hearing distance of the music could accommodate about two hundred and fifty thousand youngsters, those who could not hear did not disrupt those who could. Those who had, shared with those who didn't. And those who were needed, provided assistance. While the festival had more than its share of misfortune, those attending reacted with patience, understanding and acceptance.

Quite to the contrary as has been reported by various sources and some of the news media there were no serious health or sanitary problems at any time during the three-day weekend. Adequate sanitary facilities were provided, food was available, and medical attention was dispensed to all who may have required such assistance in the authorized locations which we had originally planned as part of the festival grounds. Problems did arise when visitors did decide to camp in unauthorized locations. These locations were not furnished with water, toilet facilities or refuse containers. Many were unaware that such facilities did in fact exist.

Due to a lack of posted signs and poor communication certain privies were
under utilized while others were overused and still others were not used
at all throughout the entire weekend. Mr. William Reynolds of the Johnny-
On-The-Spot Corporation made a valiant effort at servicing the over 300
units furnished by his company but he like everyone else had insurmountable
problems. He was able to service those privies in the concession area and
did manage to keep them in operation throughout the weekend. In the future,
internal roads must be provided and maintained so that vital services can be
at all times kept in proper operation.

Although the water supply storage tanks never went below the one quarter
level (approximately 12,000 gallons) we had a number of people who went without water. The number of spigots available were insufficient for the amount
of people attending the festival. The fact that the roads were inaccessible
prevented us from securing additional materials necessary to expand the original system. We did supplement our water supply by means of four converted
milk tankers having a capacity of approximately 5000 gallons each. The
tankers were located in areas of heavy use and were filled from the storage
tanks. The difficulty in transporting these tankers from one location to
another necessitated their being placed in locations of relative accessibility.
Complicating matters were the two heavy rainstorms (the first occurring late
Friday night and the second on Sunday afternoon) which turned the pastures
of Yasgur's Farm into a field of mud. This further prevented the moveability
of the water tankers.

The combination of overcrowding and muddy surface conditions proved highly
detrimental to our proposed plans for solid refuse collection and disposal.
The pick-up trucks were unable to make their regular collections and a large
amount of refuse, mostly consisting of paper and papergood products, began
to accumulate. Substantially less than the 300 proposed refuse receptacles
were provided. Mounds of refuse were in evidence where the participates of
the festival piled their trash and rubbish. Generally the refuse was placed
in specified locations-until the heavy rains and wind storm of Sunday afternoon at which time refuse became strewn throughout the festival site. Effective refuse collection was carried out in the concession area due to its
accessibility and proximity to the low density compacting unit. Regular collections were made and the area was policed until such time as the ground
became too muddy to do so. Refuse collection and disposal was continued
after completion of the festival weekend to the point where the festival site
is now almost entirely free of refuse. There was an accumulation of refuse
along the major arteries feeding the site, but through a dedicated effort by
Mr. Mayer Berman, Resident Engineer, and his men of the New York State Department of Transportation, cleanup operations were begun almost immediately
and within a week's time the public roads, notably Route 17B, were cleared
of all refuse.

Detailed reports of the four areas of responsibility - Water Supply, Food
Service, Sanitary Waste and Refuse are as follows:

WATER SUPPLY

Attached are the results of laboratory analyses run on samples collected
from various sources of water which were in use at the Aquarian Exposition

during August 15th through the 18th. Out of a series of 12 samples collected for bacterial analysis 2 were positive and one sample was of questionable quality. One of the positive samples was collected from well #1 on the 16th of August during a period when the well chlorinator was out of operation. This chlorinator was put back into operation shortly after the sample was collected. The other positive sample and the questionable sample were collected from a tap immediately following filtration and chlorination. These samples had not received adequate contact time since the chlorine had been in contact with the samples for less than a minute.

It should be brought out that a second sample collected from well #1 on August 16th indicated a water of safe sanitary quality at the time of sampling. Similarly all samples collected from the storage tanks which were approximately 15 minutes up the main from the point of chlorination and filtration indicated water of safe sanitary quality at the time of sampling.

Two samples for physical and chemical analysis were collected, one of raw water and one of the filtered lake water. The raw water sample indicated a highly colored and turbid water with a slight vegetable odor. The analysis also indicated a soft water with corrosive characteristics. The ammonia concentration was high and this is attributed to forest drainage into the surface supply. The nitrites and nitrates were higher than desirable and represented the initial and final product of the biochemical oxidation of ammonia respectively. The iron concentration was higher than desirable.

The physical and chemical analysis of the treated water indicated a marked reduction in color and turbidity which brought both of these physical characteristics within the acceptable limits of Part 72 of the State Sanitary Code. Significant reductions in the concentration of iron, manganese, ammonia, nitrites and nitrates were also accomplished.

The water supply facilities consisted of two high rate sand and gravel swimming pool filters supplied and operated by Clearwater Pool Supplies, Inc. of South Fallsburg, New York. These filters were followed by chlorination and furnished approximately 259,000 gals. of water a day to four (4) 12,000 gallon storage tanks located on top of a hill behind the food concession area. A detention time of approximately 15 minutes was achieved through the two 3" mains connecting the filters to the storage tanks. The lowest water level in the storage tanks observed during the three days was about one-quarter of the tank heights or 12,000 gals. of available water.

In addition to the filtered lake water, 4 well supplies were used. These wells were located in the proposed campground areas and supplied water to spigot stations for drinking, cooking and washing purposes. These wells were all about 300' deep and all except well #4 were chlorinated during use. Well #4 was not chlorinated, however, it was equipped with a sanitary well seal and the results of laboratory analysis of a sample collected from this source indicated a water of safe sanitary quality at time of sampling.

The supply was further augmented by four McBride milk tank trucks which each held approximately 5000 gals. of chlorinated water. These trucks were parked in areas which had not been originally planned for camping but which had turned overnight into major campgrounds.

- 4 -

The problems which were encountered with the water supply operations were mainly broken mains and spigots due to poor installation and choice of materials. These breaks caused temporary shut downs of sections of the distribution system and unnecessary wasting of water. The operation of the chlorinators was a problem since many of the campers were organic and objected to the chlorination of the water. These persons or other curious persons apparently were responsible for tampering with or turning off the chlorinators.

The major problems pertaining to distribution of water were that many persons had camped in areas not intended for camping and well removed from watering points. The distance these people had to carry water encouraged them to consume water of unknown quality from nearby streams, ponds and springs. In addition to this it is felt that more distribution points would have been desirable since they would have cut down on the waiting time at watering points.

Based upon the experience and observation of the members of this office the following recommendations are offered for consideration:

1. A series of small independent systems offers more insurance of continued service than does one large communal, storage and distribution system.

2. All facilities are to be installed and in working operation a minimum of fifteen days prior to the beginning of the festival.

3. The distribution system should be properly designed and installed to provide for an ease of expansion and a continuity of service. Adequate intermediate valves, sufficient distribution points and piping flexible enough to withstand the abuse of extremely heavy use, should all be incorporated within the design.

FOOD SERVICE

Food For Love, Inc. operated the main concession area which consisted of six ice cream stands which sold prepackaged ice cream products, eight soda distribution stands which sold canned soda, four food stands which sold prepackaged sandwiches, hot dogs, hamburgers, soda, half pint containers of milk and juices, and four special stands which sold fruit, cigarettes, cotton candy and script money for purchasing food at the other stands.

The food storage area was set up and maintained in a clean and orderly manner. The temperatures of the refrigerated trucks with perishable foods were checked every six hours and were found to be below 50 degrees at all times. Freezer trucks were maintained at temperatures below 10 degrees. Sandwiches came prepackaged and were delivered in refrigerated trucks. As the food stands required additional sandwiches they were transferred from the trucks to the stands. At the food stands the sandwiches were not kept under refrigeration but due to the large turnover, this did not present any serious problems.

- 5 -

A cafeteria was set up in the vicinity of the stage area for the performers and personnel of Woodstock Ventures, Inc. It appeared to be operated in a sanitary manner. They served mainly cold plates, sandwiches and box lunches. The box lunches were prepared by Horn and Hardart, Inc.

Located in a section of the campsite area known as the "Hog Farm" a kitchen was set up for the benefit of those people who could not afford to buy food and would, therefore, have had to go hungry. The food was prepared and distributed by a group calling themselves "Hog Farmers". This food, supplied by Woodstock Ventures, Inc. consisted mainly of fruits, vegetables and grains. Small amounts of eggs, milk and meat were also furnished. The sanitary conditions of the "free food" operation were not ideal, but since most of the items served were not perishable no serious health problems developed. Approximately 10,000 people per day were served by the communal people of the "Hog Farm".

Several small food vendors most notably pizza, chinese food, and soft ice cream wagons gained entrance to the festival site without inspection. This was brought to the attention of Mr. Lee Howard, Partner in Food for Love, Inc., without very much success. They continued to do business until they sold out their wares. The pizza wagons in particular were not maintaining satisfactory sanitary practices due to the large volume of business being generated. The food was not properly stored and handled, nor was it adequately prepared. And with so great a demand the food was not cooked for a sufficient period of time. In the future all food vendors should be inspected and approved by the State Health Department before being permitted access to the festival grounds. Once allowed on the premises they should be periodically inspected and if violations are not corrected, they should be closed down immediately.

Several problems were noted in the concession area. Among the more common were eating and smoking by the employees while working in the food stands. This condition could have been improved with better supervision. There were no hand washing facilities for use by food handlers after using toilets, as had been originally agreed upon. Water supply to the food stands was disrupted several times due to broken water mains, and policing the area for papers became impossible after the heavy rains produced an extensive mud problem throughout the concession area.

It is recommended that the State Health Department have complete control over all phases of the food service program including planning, inspection and enforcement in any future festival of this type. Failure to comply with Part 14 of the State Sanitary Code should bring about immediate action to close down the establishment, or that part of the establishment which is in violation of the Code. Furthermore, adequate restricted roads must be provided in order that food deliveries can be made as they are needed.

SANITARY WASTE

The toilet facilities proposed and provided for the Festival area were of the chemical toilet type and were furnished from two sources. Inspections, maintenance, scavenger service and ultimate disposal of the waste was also provided by the supplier of the toilets.

Johnny-on-the-Spot, portable chemical toilets of New York City, New York provided 30 of his big John units and had 10 more units available as standby.

Therefore, there were actually on Saturday and Sunday, 15 and 16 of August 1969, 40 Big John units available for use. The Big John unit consisted of 10 individual and separate toilet spaces, one 5 place urinal and a 900 gal. holding tank which is accessible from any of the stools or a port on the end of the unit.

Port-O-San Chemical toilets of Kearny, New Jersey furnished 250 single units which in addition to the Johnny-on-the-Spot units provided a total toilet facility of 650 stools and 200 urinal spaces. These facilities were distributed along the roads within the festival area for ease of maintenance. The preplanned camping areas, entertainment area and concession area received the benefit of these facilities. These facilities were intended for use by some 60,000 persons and were not available to the outlying unauthorized camping areas.

The disposal of waste from these units was to have been on the property of Mr. Hyman Lyman some 3 miles from the Festival area. The disposal siste was quite satisfactory in that it was accessible from a paved road, well removed from all residences, the soil was sandy, the surface of the ground water was over 15' vertically from the lowest disposal elevation, and there was no possibility of surface runoff into surface waters. There were at least five trucks provided for removal of the waste, however, their efforts were hampered by the traffic congestion and much of the waste was buried on the Festival grounds.

The major problems encountered within this area was servicing of the toilets and overnight growth of camping areas which did not have access to the toilet facilities.

The servicing of the toilets was hindered by congested roads which at times were impassable due to stalled cars and throngs of people. In addition to congestion the mud greatly reduced the scavenger trucks mobility once they left the hard road surfaces.

Observation of these facilities during the Festival lead to these comments:

1. That the multiple units such as the Big John are desirable since they can be serviced more rapidly and provide service to more persons.

2. Units similar to those discussed above should be located in areas where service will not be interrupted.

3. The disposal of waste should be in an acceptable location as close to the area of origin as possible.

4. Positive supervision of camping should be encouraged to insure that camp grounds develop where facilities have been provided.

- ·7 -

SOLID REFUSE

On July 30, 1969 Woodstock Ventures, Inc. signed a contract with the New
York Carting Company to supply equipment and manpower for the collection
and disposal of the solid waste produced during the festival. Also ar-
rangments were made with the Town of Bethel to use the Town Sanitary Land-
fill site for solid waste disposal.

The New York Carting Company agreed to supply the following items:

     One B104 stationary compactor
     Two 50 cubic yard compactor containers
     One 50 cubic yard open container (canvas covered)
     Two Roll-off 24 ft. hoists
     One mobile compactor 30 cubic yard loadmaster
     One maintenance pick-up service vehicle
     One supervisor
     Two chauffeurs and 1 relief standby
     Three hundred receptacle stands and holders
     Twenty thousand paper-can bags (or equal)
     Fifteen professional steel staplers

Although no specific count was made of the above items, it appeared that all
items were present. This equipment was deemed sufficient by all concerned
to service upwards of 50,000 people.

The 300 stand holders attached four to a post and fitted with the paper-can
bags were scattered throughout the festival site. The posts were not placed
down sufficiently deep into the ground and many fell over when loaded. The
collection points placed in the actual entertainment area were soon overflowing and merely became rubbish piles. Officials of Woodstock promised that an
additional 30 full time sanitary employees and 200 part-time employees would
be retained to pick up refuse with two pickup trucks. The two pickup trucks
were on the site but the pickup crews were never in evidence in the numbers
promised. The crews on the trucks seemed to have very little incentive to
do a proper job. Turnaround time with the small cargoes of the trucks was
very short. The trucks would have done a better job if their cargo volumes
had been increased by building up the sides of the trucks.

The 30 cubic yard loadmaster concentrated its efforts on the food concession
area but could not maneuver well after the rains turned the area into a
quagmire.

The roads throughout the festival site were blocked by spectators and spectators' vehicles, therefore, preventing refuse collection in outlying areas.
The pickup trucks brought their loads to the compactor which did an effective
job of compacting the refuse into the 50 cubic yard containers. The containers were then loaded on trailers and brought to the Bethel Sanitary Land-
fill site whenever the roads were negotiable.

On Sunday, after the heavy rain, numerous piles of rubbish were set ablaze
by the fairgoers to warm up and dry out. This resulted in pillars of gray
smoke in the area.

The following recommendations are offered for consideration at this time:

1. A greater number of pick-up trucks or small compactor trucks
   would have eased the overwhelming rubbish problem. These
   smaller vehicles would have been better abled to maneuver
   throughout the throngs of people and parked automobiles.

2. The fact that roads became inaccessible, prevented collection
   of rubbish in the more remote areas. Roads must be kept
   cleared and open for use by service and emergency vehicles.

3. A sufficient number of men must be employed to effectively
   operate a collection and disposal system. A schedule must
   be set up and strictly adhered to.

4. Sturdier garbage holder posts, properly installed should be
   required. Delivery and installation should be well in advance of the beginning of the festival in order to eliminate
   the last minute state of mass confusion.

5. Consideration might be given to the use of large "Dempsey
   Dumper" type rubbish containers, strategically located on
   the site, with a heavy concentration located behind the concession area.

6. Careful planning and better placement of the refuse receptacles,
   so as to locate them in areas of heavy use, would be most effective. Receptacles should be concentrated in those areas of
   maximum use and should be conveniently and quickly serviceable.

It is the considered opinion of this office that measures might have been
taken which would have substantially relieved many of the problems that we
encountered over the festival weekend. It is with this in mind that we offer
the following suggestions and recommendations:

1. Strict controls limiting the number of tickets to be sold to
   that planned for in the original design. The number of tickets needed to break even should be determined. All ticket
   outlets should be known and periodical reports on tickets
   sales should be submitted.

2. Adequate and restricted roadways both internally and externally
   to be used by official and emergency vehicles must be provided.
   These roads must be kept open and cleared of all pedestrians.
   A network of walkways linking all sections of the festival
   area should be constructed. These walkways would relieve the
   congested roads and allow vital facilities to be serviced and
   maintained.

3. Off-the-site parking facilities with a means of mass transportation between the parking lots and the festival grounds should
   be provided. Separate roads leading directly to the camping

grounds should be kept open for those who intend to camp out for the weekend. Law enforcement agencies directing traffic should keep the flow of traffic moving either to the parking lots or to the campsite areas.

4. All facilities should be installed on the festival site and in working operation a minimum of fifteen days prior to the opening of the festival.

5. Complete and absolute control over all food services including all individual and private concessionaires operating on the festival site. Insure compliance with the State Sanitary Code on all food handling matters.

6. An organizational chart listing all executive personnel and their specific functions and areas of responsibility must be established and submitted with their original proposal.

7. A communications system should be created with direct connections between the various agencies participating in the regulation of the festival activities. Communications between the promoters and those attending the festival should also be improved. Telephones, signs, public address announcements, ballons as well as other devices should be used in order to inform those present of the locations of the various facilities available. Conferences between the promoters and the regulating agencies should be held on a regularly scheduled basis throughout the festival weekend.

8. All system should be so designed as to allow for flexibility and expansion to meet any unexpected demands. Supplies of additional materials should be readily available for immediate delivery to the festival site. A professional maintenance crew shall be available on a 24 hour schedule during the festival, for the express purpose of making emergency repairs.

9. Adequate office space, sleeping quarters and means of transportation shall be made available for personnel of the State Health Department and all other agencies whose services may be required on a 24 hour basis.

Inspection and supervision by personnel of the New York State Health Department included the following areas of responsibility, of which primary concern was directed towards securing compliance by Woodstock Ventures, Inc. with the rules and regulations of the State Sanitary Code.

PRIVIES

1. Need of service

2. Paper

3. Structural defects

4. Handwashing facilities (soap, towels & water)

GROUNDS

    1. General police

    2. Safety hazards

REFUSE

    1. Need for pickup

    2. Operation of disposal site

FOOD SERVICE

    1. Storage of food

    2. Flies

    3. Refuse disposal

    4. Refrigeration - keep temperature record

    5. Cleanliness of food service personnel

    6. Waste disposal

WATER SUPPLY

    1. Sample from each supply twice a day

    2. Operation of equipment

    3. Check on chlorinator operation every ±4 hours. Keep records

    4. Check storage for reserve

    5. Keep pump records

    6. Keep eye on lake for swimmers
      No swimming

HANDWASHING FACILITIES

    1. Soap, towels and water

Special acknowledgement and acclaim should be bestowed on those persons whose contribution and efforts in a time of near crisis, prevented a major disaster from materializing. These men who gave unhesitatingly of their time and energies deserve the accolades of all concerned for without their contributions the results would have most certainly been disasterous. To enumerate on their praiseworthy accomplishments would require a report twice this size. Suffice it to say that these dedicated men did what had to be done and did it in a highly professional manner. All the people of Sullivan County are extremely thankful that men of their calibre were available on that very eventful weekend.

Sullivan County Sheriff Louis Ratner - who was responsible for coordinating the efforts of all the agencies involved.

State Health Department Planning Consultant Mr. R. Mattox - whose on-site assistance, especially in the first aid station, was of primary importance.

District Health Officer Dr. M. Lipari - whose guidance and advice were most instrumental in planning and supervising the festival.

Regional Engineer Mr. A. Baskous - whose on-site observations and recommendations proved most helpful to us in the performance of our duties.

Superintendent of Monticello Central School System Dr. Ruttiger - who organized the Monticello food and medical programs which provided assistance to hungry and sick youths.

Monticello Chief of Police Mr. L. Yank - who maintained law and order in the Village of Monticello without a single incident throughout the prolonged weekend.

Assistant ~~District~~ General Attorney for Sullivan County Mr. M. Cohen - who provided valuable legal assistance and guidance.

Department of Transportation Resident Engineer Mr. M. Berman - whose efforts in clearing Rt. 17B of traffic and afterwards of debris were outstanding.

Department of Agriculture and Markets representative Mr. H. Berlin - who supervised and inspected food services, food handling and food preparation.

Consulting Engineer for Woodstock Ventures, Inc. Mr. B. Lueck, P.E. - who acted as liason between the State Health Department and Woodstock Ventures overseeing all engineering phases.

Clearwater Swimming Pool representative Mr. B. Kegan - who kept the water supply filter system in operation throughout the weekend by working 24 hours a day.

Johnny-On-The-Spot representative Mr. W. Reynolds - who made a supreme effort in servicing the toilet facilities.

State Health Department representatives Mr. T. Allen, Mr. J. Kwak and Mr. W. Krusanocker - who provided constant surveillance, guidance, advice and assistance throughout the planning and presentation of this festival. They were essential in overseeing that the facilities were kept in proper operation throughout the festival weekend.

3. C.B. Esselstyn, M.D., Director of Emergency Medical Services, New York State Department of Health; reports to New York State Department of Health, August 19, 1969.

New York State Department of He
Albany Regional Office
Taxation and Finance Bldg. (#9)
Room 412
State Office Building Campus
Albany, New York 12226

August 19, 1969

Doctor Mahedy - Medical Services

Doctor Esselstyn - Emergency Medical Services

Folk Song Festival in Bethel, New York, August 15, 16 and 17

Plans for the public health aspects of this gathering were submitted and reviewed by Doctor McMahon's office. They were found to be adequate for the estimated 50,000, who were expected to attend.

Arrangements had been made by the promoters to cover the possible ambulance needs through a contract with the Sullivan County commercial ambulance company in Monticello with five vehicles. To make sure that coverage was in order Dr. Norbert Shay was dispatched and reviewed the ambulance situation Friday, August 15, 1969.

Arrangements for medical services had been made with a team of physicians under the direction of Dr. William Abruzzi of Wappingers Falls together with a supply of nurses.

On Sunday morning, August 1?, I received a call from Mr. Ray Darbuti that there was a desperate need for additional ambulances. Although ambulances were available at Camp Smith, General O'Hara canceled the request.

At this stage I contacted Mr. Max Yasgur, owner of the property where the festival was being held. Mr. Yasgur has an extensive milk route and volunteered to make some of his milk trucks available which might be used to carry litters. Shortly after this Mr. Yasgur called me back saying that he had been in touch with Mr. Genung who was in charge of security who told him that there was no need for ambulances.

In order to evaluate the situation I went to the Monticello Office of Civil Defense and from there went to the Monticello School where an emergency hospital had been

New York State Department of Health
Albany Regional Office
Taxation and Finance Bldg. (#9)
Room 412
State Office Building Campus
Albany, N.

New York State Department of Health
Albany Regional Office
Taxation and Finance Bldg. (#9)
Room 412
State Office Building Campus
Albany, New York 12226

Doctor Mahady   -2-   August 19, 1969

established with the benefit of a 100 cots and blankets obtained
from the Medical Defense Stockpile. From there I took a
helicopter which had been dispatched from Stewart Air Force Base
to the scene of the festival where I spent the rest of the
afternoon evaluating developments. There obviously was no need
for more ambulances. Two helicopters had been dispatched from
Stewart Air Force Base at the request of the Sheriff of Sullivan
County and on the preceding day when cases had begun to accumulate
at the improvised hospital in the field, they were able to drain
off the excessive load which was over and beyond that which
could be transported by the Sullivan County ambulances which were
seriously compromised because of blocked roads.

Actually I felt that the medical coverage was well
organized under the direction of Dr. William Abruzzi. There
were 11 first aid stations manned by nurses scattered throughout the landscape. Of these, one was covered by a psychiatric
team composed of two psychiatrists and another by a psychiatric
social worker. Cases were triaged at these areas and if
necessary brought to the hospital tent which had been set up at
the field. Triage at this point forwarded the more seriously
involved into the hospital which had been set up at the school
at Monticello. From here if necessary they were referred to
surrounding hospitals. The local hospitals rapidly became filled
and cases were subsequently taken as far as Middletown. Certain
other cases were taken directly from the field hospital to local
hospitals.

The bulk of the emergencies consisted of those suffering
from heat exhaustion, "bad trips", burns mostly from lighter
fluid which had been applied to charcoal campfires, cuts mostly
on barefoot, bruises, epilepsy which was surprisingly prominent
and two or three hot bellies. In addition two girls went into
labor.

The supplies which became short were for nalline, valium,
dilantin, tetanus toxoid and sanitary napkins of all varieties.

The most obvious public health hazard was the accumulation
of piles of garbage which were beginning to smell in the hot
sun which appeared between showers. Doctor McMahon was notified
but already aware of the problem.

I believe the inflexibility of mobilizing Medical
Defense resources should be reviewed and am recommending to
General Asensio that a critique be held by those involved as soon

as possible while memories are fresh in order to document those
things that might be learned by this experience. In the meantime we are gathering statistics from Sullivan Ambulance and
Doctor Abruzzi.

This was a good demonstration of the importance of
the use of helicopters for inaccessible situations. It also
demonstrated that helicopters can be made available when
needed through existing resources.

In spite of the emergency which was created by the
overwhelming, unexpected number, I believe the health problems
were handled expeditiously. The cooperative spirit and orderly
conduct of this mass of humanity facilitated the overworked
skeleton medical team.

New York State Department of Health
Albany Regional Office
Taxation and Finance Bldg. (#9)
Room 412
State Office Building Campus
Albany, New York 12226

CBE/pf
cc: Mr. O'Neill
    Mr. Handi

4. C.B. Esselstyn, M.D., Director of Emergency Medical Services, New York State Department of Health; reports to New York State Department of Health, September 8, 1969 ("Thomas MacFarland" refers to Thomas McFarlin).

New York State Department of Health
Albany Regional Office
Taxation and Finance Bldg. (#9)
Room 412
State Office Building Campus
Albany, New York 12203

September 8, 1969 RECEIVED

Dr. Caldwell B. Esselstyn

SEP 9 1969

Dr. Norbert J. Shay

N.Y. STATE DEPT. OF HEALTH
ALBANY REGIONAL OFFICE

Return visit to Monticello following "Happening" at White Lake

I went to Monticello on Thursday, August 21st for a follow-up talk after the "Music and Peace Festival" at White Lake.

The week-end was discussed in some detail with Mr. Thomas MacFarland, owner of the Sullivan County Ambulance Service (Commercial). His initial contract with Woodstock Ventures, Inc. was for $600.00 to provide two ambulances on the grounds 24-hours a day for the three days of the festival. The crowd began arriving a day early so he was asked to provide ambulance coverage beginning on Thursday rather than Friday and he remained on the grounds until Tuesday and provided four ambulances. Because of the modified contract he was given a check for $2,300 but as of August 21st had not cashed it because Woodstock Ventures, Inc. asked him to please call them before cashing it. This contract was to pick sick and injured victims up on the grounds and bring them to the tent hospital plus bringing serious emergencies to area hospitals.

Tom said another commercial ambulance service was hired, without his knowledge, for a period of 24 hours. This service took two calls and they saw no more of them after that. It is very possible this was Sloper-Willen Ambulance Service, Inc. of Wappinger Falls. However, I am not at all sure. This service is not registered with the Bureau as an Invalid Coach or otherwise.

Sullivan County Ambulance Service sustained $2800 worth of damages to their ambulances during the event. The damage consisted of burned-out transmissions, cut tires and things of that nature. Woodstock Ventures has promised to pay for these damages as soon as money is available.

On Thursday, the 14th of August there were no doctors available on the grounds. His attendants performed necessary first-aid and were able to bring victims to area hospitals. Just before noon on Friday the 15th it became impossible to move patients by land ambulance of the grounds. However, about this point two doctors arrived and two helicopters were available to transport victims. Later of course more doctors and medical supplies were flown in. All his own supplies were used up early in the game, however, he was able to replenish them from supplies flown into tent hospital, etc. He did make one helicopter trip for more oxygen.

New York State Department of Health
Albany Regional Office

Albany Regional Office
Taxation and Finance Bldg. (#
Room 412
State Office Building Campus
Albany, New York 12226

The Liberty Volunteer Ambulance Service was there with their
ambulance but that left Liberty without ambulance service. Volunteers
from other neighboring communities were on the grounds helping wherever
they could but they left their ambulances home to cover their own areas.

Mr. MacFarland gave a lot of credit to the so-called "Hog Farmers."
He said they performed first-aid, handled communications, counseled those
in trouble (particularly those high on drugs), cleaned up and made themselves generally available for any help they could be. Tom stressed the
politeness, peace, serenity and the general willingness to help of the
entire gathering. He said at no time was an ambulance of his stuck in the
mud for more than five minutes. It was noted that at no time did he have
to administer first-aid to a patient for injury resulting from violence or
fights of any nature. The hog farmers did ask him not to use his siren if
he could avoid it because they found for some reason or other this would
turn them on.

He complained that where the hospitals were located on the grounds
it was rather difficult getting an ambulance to them. They had to be
extremely careful driving over the fields to pick up victims as people were
lying all over under blankets, in sleeping bags, etc.

He noted there was a shortage of gasoline for helicopters and
ambulances. It was also mentioned that Dr. Abruzzi got very excited at
times and it was difficult to understand him over the radio.

Mr. MacFarland said he handled well over three hundred calls altogether.
These included picking victims up on the grounds and taking them to the tent
hospital, taking patients from tent hospital to helicopters, bringing patients
from the grounds to area hospitals and also shuttling serious cases from the
school in Monticello to nearby hospitals. Initially he started logging calls
but this became impossible as it did with switchboard and telephone answering
service operators. He may be able to get some compensation from the County
for shuttling patients from temporary hospital in the school to area hospitals.

I talked with one of the County Supervisors, Mr. Ralph Meyer. He
spoke very highly of the Sullivan County Ambulance Service and said they did
an excellent job under the circumstances.

Mr. MacFarland had several suggestions:

1. In the event something like this is repeated he strongly suggested
that a briefing meeting be held before hand. The meeting should be attended
by medical and para-medical people, hospital representatives, police, fire,
Sheriff's department, State Troopers, County Supervisors, etc. All eventuali-
ties should be discussed and definite plans made. He hinted at the formation
of an Emergency Medical Care Council without any prodding from me.

2. He strongly suggests that disaster drills be held both announced
and unannounced. They should involve the hospitals, ambulance services, fire
departments, law enforcement agencies, medical and para-medical personnel, etc

5. Abbie Hoffman, "Survival Sheet."

W ome to Hip City, USA. We' re ne of the largest cities i:
f: ica (population 300,000 a (r wing all the time). We've go t
7   : . :   : l. hwir :m   . . traffic death, 15 miscarriages
an a lot of mud. This is a d at r area.

    ore we go from here. depen on all of us. The people who promoted
th s festival have been ver lu by their own creation. We can no
lo er remain passive consume. / w have to begin to fend for ourselves.

ACCESS -- The highways leadin to he festival site are now blocked .
Cars are being bturned back i: an ffort to clear highway 17B. The
best thing you can do is to s y u til the roads are cleared. If you
de ide to split and get stuck a team of repairmen is cruising the
area and will free your car. n't leave your vehicle.

S NITATION -- Please stay off he oads. Garbage trucks need clear
rights-of-way to pick up tras. Ei her burn your trash or dump it
IN BAGS along the road (look r t e stands with green bags hanging
from them.) You MUST clean yo a a to avoid a severe health hazard.

M DICAL -- There are two majo medical stations. Minor stuff (cuts,
b ses) can be taken care of t the SOUTH STATION near the Hog Farm,
s ious injuries will be tree d t the health trailer at the MAIN
I RSECTION, and drug freake s will be tended by the Hog Farm (red
o   and) people at the SOUTH UN ROUND.
  planeload of doctors are ing airlifted from New York City, and
a eet of helicopters is bei g gathered to drop medical supplies.
 y trained medical person t ould report to the above medical
c   ers.
   not take any light blue lat acid and understand that taking
   ng dope at this time may ike you a drag in a survival situation.
   n't run naked in the hot sn or any period of time. Water blisters
c painful.

W ER -- Water is scarce. Sha e and conserve all water. Do not drink
w er unless it is crystal-cl ar. Check with festival and Hog Farm
p ple before using any open ing mains. New mains are being readied.
W will announce their locat as hen they are made available. Black
a d white pipes are water pip s, on't use for walking or bridges.
 ey break easily.
  The lake is now a main sou e o water. Swimming will ruin the
 urification system -- think wic before taking a dip.

FOOD -- You should not be pig ish about your food and water. As
with medicine, festival peop ha e promised that food will be
airlifted into the area. The o. arm will continue to serve meals
i the SOUTH AREA.

VOLUNTEERS -- Go to info. st d a main intersection

G NERAL HINTS - The thing t d s survive and share. Organize
  r own camping area so tha e c yone makes it through uncomfortable
  es ahead. Figure out what wi ust do and the best ways to get it done.

   OPLE WHO CAN HELP DISTRIBU l G SS LEAFLET SHOULD COME TO THE MOVEMENT
   TY AREA IN TE SOUTH CAMP(VU II .
   D AND PAS ON

6. Dr. Dombeck letter

RICHARD J. MALLOY   173

Nov 5 19 85   50-547/219

Pay to the order of Dr. Sol Dombeck $ 25—

Twenty Five and xx/100 ———   DOLLARS

STATE EMPLOYEES FEDERAL
CREDIT UNION
P.O. BOX 1218V, ALBANY, N.Y. 12212

Richard J. Malloy

Dear Dr. Dombeck

Enclosed please find my check in the amount of $25

This is for services rendered and in appreciation of the help you gave me at the Woodstock festival. At that time you treated a badly cut foot (mine) and also fed a very hungry person (me.)

Why it took me 16 years to keep a promise and get in touch with you regarding settlement of a bill, (I had no money and promised to get in touch about payment), is a long and inexcusable story, which I won't bore you with. I never forgot your help, I just never bothered to pay.

Please accept both my check and my apology.

Sincerely

Richard J. Malloy

7. New York State Department of Health, "Permit to Operate a Temporary Residence"

PERMIT
TO OPERATE A TEMPORARY RESIDENCE

YASGUR FARM # 5 - MAX YASGUR

the operator of a temporary residence known as

Mel Lawrence - Woodstock Ventures Inc.

located in the

Town of Bethel in Sullivan County

is granted this permit to operate the above-named temporary residence, as provided by Part 7 of the Sanitary Code, established by the Public Health Council of the State of New York.

This permit will expire upon the date specified below or upon a change of the operator. It is not transferable or assignable. It may be revoked as provided in the Sanitary Code. It shall be posted or kept on file and made available by the operator on request. This permit is granted subject to any and all State, local and municipal laws, ordinances, codes, rules and regulations.

Signature of Issuing Officer ....*Michael Lifari*..........................

Title District Health Officer

Department New York State Department of Health

Address 6 Prince Street, Monticello, New York

Date of Issuance: August 4, 1969

Date of Expiration: September 1, 1969

Form San. 143 (Rev. 12/66)

8. Wesley A. Pomeroy, Security Consultant, Woodstock Ventures, Inc.
Page 3 of his security plan, "Aquarian Festival" Bethel, New York,
August 15, 16 & 17, 1969

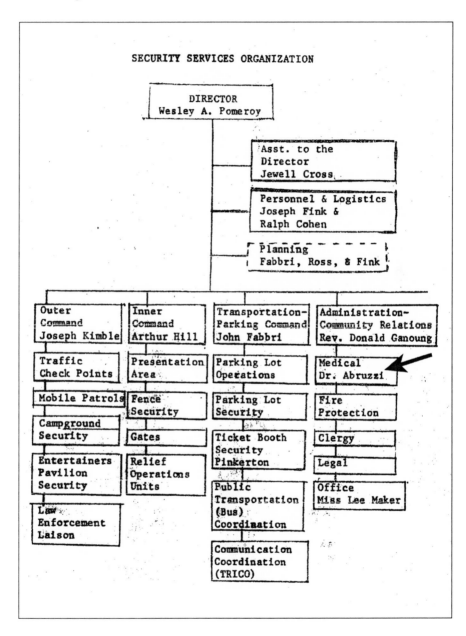

9. Sullivan County Ambulance Service.

Sullivan County Ambulance Service was the only commercial service in Sullivan County in 1969 and had a contract to provide ambulance services at the Woodstock Festival. Below: Their 1963 Superior Cadillac Rescuer in action at the festival.

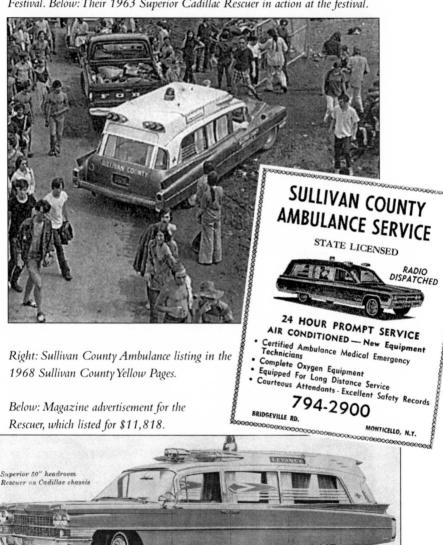

Right: Sullivan County Ambulance listing in the 1968 Sullivan County Yellow Pages.

Below: Magazine advertisement for the Rescuer, which listed for $11,818.

SULLIVAN COUNTY AMBULANCE SERVICE

STATE LICENSED

RADIO DISPATCHED

24 HOUR PROMPT SERVICE
AIR CONDITIONED — New Equipment
- Certified Ambulance Medical Emergency Technicians
- Complete Oxygen Equipment
- Equipped For Long Distance Service
- Courteous Attendants - Excellent Safety Records

794-2900

BRIDGEVILLE RD.   MONTICELLO, N.Y.

Superior 50" headroom Rescuer on Cadillac chassis

SUPERIOR FOR 1963

10. Mobilemedic 51-93 (2008 American Emergency Vehicles, Type II).

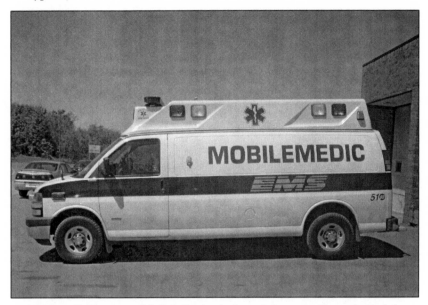

Mobilemedic Emergency Medical Services is the ambulance provider at the Bethel Woods Center for the Arts, which is on the site of the 1969 Woodstock Festival. Mobilemedic has provided Advanced Life Support ambulance services in Sullivan County since 1991.

11. The Musuem at Bethel Woods Center for the Arts

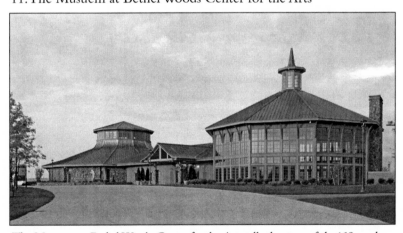

The Museum at Bethel Woods Center for the Arts tells the story of the '60s and Woodstock at the site of the 1969 Woodstock Festival.

12. Max Yasgur's statement about the 1969 Woodstock Music Festival.

Bethel, Monday August 18, 1969

Max Yasgur, owner of the farm rented by the Woodstock Arts Festival promoters issued the following statement Monday afternoon:

Three weeks ago the citizens of Wallkill, New York banished from their community a group of young people seeking three days of music and peace. In desperation, looking for a site on which to hold their festival, Woodstock Ventures came to Bethel. For 2 weeks it rained daily while the young people toiled around the clock in an almost impossible effort to turn hay fields into a festival site. A playground was constructed for children, complete with animals, miles of chain link fence was erected, a magnificent stage was built, five wells were drilled, electric service was brought in from five miles away, thousands of portable toilets were positioned and generally every effort possible was made to handle a maximum expected turnout of 50,000 people per day.

The young people who built Aquarian began allaying the fears of the local people with whom they had contact. They were industrious, polite and policed up after themselves.

On the eve of the festival, however, adults and nature combined to form a severe test of pressure and problems for the Aquarian Festival. New York City Police Commissioner, Howard Leary prevented an estimated 350 off-duty police from serving as security officers as they had originally been hired to do. One hundred buses which had been scheduled to shuttle in festival patrons, free of charge, from outlaying parking lots were suddenly unavailable. Then finally the rains came. So did the young people. Eight or ten times as many people came as had ever been anticipated.

Under the severe strain of almost one half million people the facilities broke down. Parking in rain soaked fields became impossible. Traffic with an understaffed security force became an impossible snarl. The wells, overtaxed, were hardly able to keep up with the demand and the sanitation facilities became inaccessible to maintenance. By the early morning hours of Saturday I feared that a major catastrophe was in the making. I tried to imagine what a population larger than Albany and perhaps as large as Buffalo might do in a situation in which they were wet, thirsty, hungry, tired and immobile and facing nothing but more of the same. The prospects were horrifying. Some had come over 3000 miles and had paid $18.00 for tickets only to find that they had to walk the last five miles in the rain to reach an over full festival site where no tickets were being collected because the management feared someone might be hurt in the crush at the gate. What would you envision that a group of a half million professional football or other sport fans might do under similar circumstances.

But, thank heaven, none of our fears were realized. What happened at Bethel this past weekend was that those young people together with our local residents turned the Aquarian Festival into a dramatic victory for the spirit of peace, good will and human kindness. Hungry youths shared everything they had. Local residents poured out to volunteer food and aid. Well meaning youths looking for a place to rest and something to eat strayed on private property built fires out of fences and slept in fields. My neighbors were magnificent. They had nothing to gain from the festival. They were not receiving rent or selling anything. They were merely trying to run their dairy farms and homes. They woke to find thousands of young people camping on their lawns and fields. Yet through it all there was not one incident, as my neighbors for whom my heart goes out more than they can know, rose to the occasion. The State Police, Sheriff Ratner and his overworked force, local police and volunteers from the surrounding community justly received the highest praise from festival goers, staff and local residents. Together they organized emergency traffic and emergency procedures that finally succeeded in bringing order out of the traffic and relief to the inundated first aid facilities. With the aid of Armed Forces helicopters and local volunteers, potential medical crises was averted. They deserve the highest possible commendation, each and every one, for the magnificent way in which they handled the situation.

I am of course exceedingly sorry for many neighbors and

friends who suffered damage. The fault, if there be one, lies simply in the fact that ten times as many youths came to the festival as had been anticipated and of course the rain then made a bad situation terrible. But damage is repairable by money and effort.

It seems evident to me that if one-half million young people came to Sullivan County there must be fifteen to twenty million of them in America. It has been estimated that 80 per cent were on some form of narcotics. Although this is merely a guess and not a proven fact, if it is so the problem is more urgent than any of us realized.

The militant groups and the communist organizers were here and nothing would have proven their point more than a riot. But they couldn't get a riot started no matter how they tried because, as the young people said, "this was a cool scene" with no reason for violence. I for one have learned a lesson I will not forget.

I realize that as a American we are talking about most of our generation of young people, many of whom are the young intelligentsia of our society. Many of them are attending college, many have graduate degrees and the one thing that they have in common is that they are all thinkers. Possibly some are impractical dreamers but all are thinkers and deeply concerned about their future and even more about the future of America and the form of government that I love.

These young people, whom my age group refer to as the "beat generation" are the voters and the lawmakers of tomorrow. If they are a "beat generation" then we, the so-called establishment, their parents, made them so. Our generation will have to decide and decide quickly whether we are going to give these young people a "fair shake" or are going to discount them because they don't cut their hair or wear their clothing the way we would like them to. If we don't listen to their gripes, the radical and extremists will and then we can and will have continued anarchy and violence in America.

It has been stated and undoubtedly grossly overstated that 80 per cent of the festival visitors were on some form of narcotics. If these figures are true it is clear that the basic problem is the climate in our country which makes such facts possible. Whether or not those who are now using drugs can be helped is primarily a medical problem, but the problem of preventing further drug use is the problem that my generation must face. If we want our young people to be free of the horrible effects of drug addiction then we must provide for them a climate in which they can grow without being forced to drugs to avoid our society.

It was proven in Bethel that these young people do not want fo follow all the radical groups that are pressuring them. In Bethel, in spite of terrible adversity one half million people remained peaceful and I believe that they and the millions of others like them, would like to become part of the peaceful society with us. But, if we don't welcome them, if we don't give them a fair shake, if we don't listen to their complaints and try to reason out the solution with them what choice will they have. The radical groups will listen to their complaints and will make efforts to help them. If we close the doors into our society they will only be left with choosing the radicals. As the late Robert F. Kennedy realized. It is with these young people that we share this nation and with them that our form of government must be run. But if we exclude them it will be our blame for having forced them to the anarchy of the radicals.

If a half million people at the Aquarian Festival could turn such adverse conditions, filled with the possibility of disaster, riot, looting and catastrophe into three days of music and peace, then perhaps there is hope that if we join with them we can turn those adversities that are the problems of America today into a hope for a brighter and more peaceful future.

In the final analysis, however, the material aspects of Aquarian, such a local loss of revenue at the track and the monumental inconvenience to local residents are far less important than the lesson that was to be learned.

Notes

~~~~~~

1 The Calm Before

[1.] Joel Makower, *Woodstock: The Oral History* (New York: Doubleday, 1989) p. 254.

[2.] Jean Young and Michael Lang, *Woodstock Festival Remembered* (New York: Ballantine, 1979) p. 30.

[3.] Joel Makower, *Woodstock: The Oral History* (New York: Doubleday, 1989), p.271.

[4.] William Abruzzi, M.D., "A White Lake Happening," report to New York State Department of Health, September 2, 1969, p. 6.

[5.] *New York Times* (August 16, 1969, p.1)`

[6.] Jean Young and Michael Lang, *Woodstock Festival Remembered* (New York: Ballantine, 1979) p. 126.

[7.] William Abruzzi, M.D., "A White Lake Happening," report to New York State Department of Health, September 2, 1969, p. 1.

[8.] Middletown, N.Y., *Times Herald-Record*, August 12, 1989, p. 12.

[9.] Joel Makower, *Woodstock: The Oral History* (New York: Doubleday, 1989), p. 65.

[10.] Gavis interview.

[11.] Interview, Lowenthal.

[12.] Bob Spitz, *Barefoot in Babylon: The Creation of the Woodstock Music Festival, 1969* (New York: Norton, 1989), p. 326.

[13.] William Abruzzi, M.D., "A White Lake Happening," report to New York State Department of Health, September 2, 1969, p. 1.

[14] New York State Department of Health, Albany Regional Office, "Environmental Health and Emergency Medical Services Report on the Woodstock Music and Art Fair (Aquarius Festival), White Lake, Bethel Town, Sullivan County, N.Y., September 25, 1969, p. 1.

[15] William Abruzzi, M.D., "A White Lake Happening," report to New York State Department of Health, September 2, 1969, p. 1.

[16] Bob Spitz, *Barefoot in Babylon: The Creation of the Woodstock Music Festival, 1969* (New York: Norton, 1989), p. 371.

[17] Ibid., p. 422.

[18] Joel Makower, *Woodstock: The Oral History* (New York: Doubleday, 1989), p. 254.

[19] Ibid., p. 255.

[20] Ibid., p. 247.

[21] Ibid., p. 257.

[22] Ibid., p. 247.

[23] Middletown, N.Y., *Times Herald-Record* (August 16, 1969).

[24] Middletown, N.Y., *Times Herald-Record* (August 12, 1989).

[25] Joel Makower, *Woodstock: The Oral History* (New York: Doubleday, 1989), p. 162.

[26] Middletown, N.Y., *Times Herald-Record* (August 9, 1969).

[27] Lisa Law, Flashing on the Sixties, (Santa Rosa: Square Books, 2000)

[28] Middletown, N.Y., *Times Herald-Record* (August 18, 1969).

[29] Personal communication, Sutton.

[30] The Medical Post (April 24, 2001).

[31] Life (August 1989).

[32] Joel Makower, *Woodstock: The Oral History* (New York: Doubleday, 1989), p. 155.

[33] Ibid., p. 261.

[34] Ibid., p. 262.

[35] Abbie Hoffman, *Woodstock Nation: A Talk-Rock Album* (New York: Vintage, 1969), p. 136.

[36] Ibid., p. 135.

[37] Sydney P. Schiff, M.D., Chief of Staff, Community General Hospital, report.

[38] Ibid.

[39] Ibid.

[40] Middletown, N.Y., *Times Herald-Record* (August 16, 1969), p. 7.

2 Into the Maelstrom

[1.] William Abruzzi, M.D., "A White Lake Happening," report to New York State Department of Health, September 2, 1969, p. 4.

[2.] Middletown, N.Y., *Times Herald-Record* (August 16, 1969).

[3.] *New York Times* (August 17, 1969, p. 80).

[4.] Toronto *Globe & Mail* (August 19, 1969).

[5.] Middletown, N.Y., *Times Herald-Record* (August 18, 1969, p. 9).

[6.] Middletown, N.Y., *Times Herald-Record* (August 16, 1969).

[7.] William Abruzzi, M.D., "A White Lake Happening," report to New York State Department of Health, September 2, 1969, p. 4.

[8.] Joel Makower, *Woodstock: The Oral History* (New York: Doubleday, 1989), p. 270.

[9.] Personal communication, Boor.

[10.] Liberty *News* (September 4, 1969).

[11.] Middletown, N.Y., *Times Herald-Record* (August 16, 1969).

[12.] Middletown, N.Y., *Times Herald-Record* (August 16, 1969).

[13.] Joel Makower, *Woodstock: The Oral History* (New York: Doubleday, 1989), p. 259.

[14.] Ibid., p. 260.

[15.] Personal communication, St. Louis.

[16.] Report, Sheriff Deputy Phillip Key.

[17.] Personal communication, Boor.

[18.] Middletown, N.Y., *Times Herald-Record* (August 18, 1969).

[19.] *New York Sunday News* (August 17, 1969) p. 3.

[20.] Ibid, p. 3.

[21.] Sydney P. Schiff, M.D., Chief of Staff, Community General Hospital, report.

[22.] Interview, Mischa Leshner.

[23.] Report, Lt. Ralph Breaky.

[24.] *New York Times* (August 18, 1969, p. 25).

[25.] Joel Makower, *Woodstock: The Oral History* (New York: Doubleday, 1989), p. 265.

[26.] Ibid., p. 265.

[27.] Ibid., p. 265.

[28.] Ibid., p. 270.

[29.] Ibid., p. 268.

[30.] Middletown, N.Y., *Times Herald-Record* (August 16, 1969).

[31.] Sydney P. Schiff, M.D., Chief of Staff, Community General Hospital, report.

[32]. Middletown, N.Y., *Times Herald-Record* (August 12, 1989), p. 27.

[33]. Ibid., p. 27.

[34]. Wavy Gravy interview.

[35]. Joel Makower, *Woodstock: The Oral History* (New York: Doubleday, 1989), p. 267.

[36]. Interview, Sebastian.

[37]. Abbie Hoffman, *Woodstock Nation: A Talk-Rock Album* (New York: Vintage, 1969), p. 138.

[38]. Joel Makower, *Woodstock: The Oral History* (New York: Doubleday, 1989), p. 264.

[39]. Ibid., p. 139.

[40]. Middletown, N.Y., *Times Herald-Record* (August 12, 1989), p. 34.

[41]. Ibid., p. 34.

[42]. Jack Curry, *Woodstock: The Summer of Our Lives* (New York: Weidenfeld & Nicolson, 1989), p. 167.

[43]. Joel Makower, *Woodstock: The Oral History* (New York: Doubleday, 1989), p. 265.

[44]. Ibid., p. 270.

[45]. Deputy Sheriff Frank Zurawski, report.

[46]. Bob Spitz, *Barefoot in Babylon: The Creation of the Woodstock ` Festival, 1969* (New York: Norton, 1989), p. 455.

[47]. Joel Makower, *Woodstock: The Oral History* (New York: Doubleday, 1989), p. 267.

[48]. Woodstock Survival Sheet, accessed March 18, 2009: http://www.geocities.com/Athens/3548/woodstock.html

[49]. Middletown, N.Y., *Times Herald-Record* (August 18, 1969).

[50]. Report, Leiber.

[51]. Middletown, N.Y., *Times Herald-Record* (August 22, 1969).

[52]. Joel Makower, *Woodstock: The Oral History* (New York: Doubleday, 1989), p. 428.

[53]. Participant memories, Bethel Woods Center for the Arts museum.

[54]. Interview, Cohen.

[55]. Port Jervis, N.Y. *Union-Gazette* (August 18, 1969).

[56]. Report, Lieber.

[57]. Lisa Law, *Flashing on the Sixties* Square Books (Santa Rosa: Square Books, 2000).

[58]. Middletown, N.Y., *Times Herald-Record* (August 22, 1969).`

[59]. Liberty *News* (September 4, 1969).

8 Health and Healing

1. Glen Joshpe, *Joshpe's Journey*, Stamford: Stonecrest Publishers, 2001.
2. Personal communication, Robert J. Flynn, March 2009.
3. Middletown, N.Y., *Times Herald-Record* (August 27, 1969).
4. Middletown, N.Y., *Times Herald-Record* (August 12, 1989).
5. Middletown, N.Y., *Times Herald-Record* (August 27, 1969).
6. Personal communication, Wexler.
7. Personal communication, Lucille Thalmann Rudiger.
8. Middletown, N.Y., *Times Herald-Record* (August 27, 1969).
9. Joel Makower, *Woodstock: The Oral History* (New York: Doubleday, 1989), p. 256.
10. Personal communication, Aprilante.
11. *New York Times* (July 1, 2006).
12. Interview, Hahn.
13. Interview, Frances Marks.
14. Interview, Pollets.
15. Middletown, N.Y., *Times Herald-Record* (August 12, 1989).
16. Interview, Rose Gerami Raimond.
17. Middletown, N.Y., *Times Herald-Record* (August 12, 1989).
18. Middletown, N.Y., *Times Herald-Record* (August 27, 1969).
19. *Life* (August 1989)
20. Personal communication, Rudiger.
21. Port Jervis, N.Y. *Union-Gazette* (August 18, 1969).
22. Joel Makower, *Woodstock: The Oral History* (New York: Doubleday, 1989), p. 258.
23. Joel Rosenman and John Roberts, *Young Men with Unlimited Capital* (New York: Harcourt Brace Jovanovich, 1974) p. 172.
24. Joel Makower, *Woodstock: The Oral History* (New York: Doubleday, 1989), p. 258.
25. Jean Young and Michael Lang, *Woodstock Festival Remembered* (New York: Ballantine, 1979), p.124.
26. Interview, Leschner.
27. Interview, Helen Reno.
28. Interview, Fried.
29. Personal communication, Lashinsky.
30. Sydney P. Schiff, M.D., Chief of Staff, Community General Hospital, report.
31. Personal communication, Dombeck.

[32.] Interview, Gavis.

[33.] Bob Spitz, *Barefoot in Babylon: The Creation of the Woodstock Music Festival,* 1969 (New York: Norton, 1989), p. 453.

[34.] Joel Makower, *Woodstock: The Oral History* (New York: Doubleday, 1989), p. 272.

[35.] *Miami Herald,* August 18, 1969.

[36.] Middletown, N.Y., *Times Herald-Record* (August 12, 1989), p. 34.

¾ A Little Heaven

[1.] Interview, Leshner.

[2.] William Abruzzi, M.D., "A White Lake Happening," report to New York State Department of Health p. 7.

[3.] Ellenville *Press* (August 21, 1969).

[4.] Interview, Pollets.

[5.] *Newsday* (August 18, 1969).

[6.] Joel Makower, *Woodstock: The Oral History* (New York: Doubleday, 1989), p. 258.

[7.] C.B. Esselstyn, M.D., Director of Emergency Medical Services, New York State Department of Health; report to New York State Department of Health, September 9, 1969.

[8.] Community General Hospital, Board of Trustees, Business Minutes September 3, 1969.

[9.] Monticello Board of Education, meeting minutes, August 19, 1969

[10.] Joel Makower, *Woodstock: The Oral History* (New York: Doubleday, 1989), p. 268.

[11.] Ibid., p. 263.

[12.] Ibid., p. 272.

[13.] Ibid., p. 260.

[14.] C.B. Esselstyn, M.D., Director of Emergency Medical Services, New York State Department of Health; report to New York State Department of Health, September 9, 1969.

[15.] Middletown, N.Y., *Times Herald-Record* (August 16, 18, 1969).

[16.] Middletown, N.Y., *Times Herald-Record* (August 18, 1969, p. 9)

[17.] Joel Makower, *Woodstock: The Oral History* (New York: Doubleday, 1989), p. 231.

[18.] Elliot Tiber, *Taking Woodstock: A True Story of a Riot, a Concert, and a Life* (Garden City Park, NY: Square One, 2007) p., 204.

19. *New York Times* (August 14, 1989).

20. Gerald Lieber, P.E., Senior Sanitary Engineer, Monticello Subdistrict, report to New York State Department of Health, September 8, 1969.

21. Ibid.

22. William Abruzzi, M.D., "A White Lake Happening," report to New York State Department of Health, September 2, 1969.

23. Personal communication, Baxter.

24. Joel Makower, *Woodstock: The Oral History* (New York: Doubleday, 1989), p. 274.

25. Ibid., p. 272.

26. Jean Young and Michael Lang, *Woodstock Festival Remembered* (New York: Ballantine, 1979), p. 126.

27. Abbie Hoffman, *Woodstock Nation: A Talk-Rock Album* (New York: Vintage, 1969), p. 102.

28. Joel Makower, *Woodstock: The Oral History* (New York: Doubleday, 1989), p. 271.

29. William Abruzzi, M.D., "A White Lake Happening," report to New York State Department of Health, September 2, 1969.

Sources

~~~~~~~~~~

Collections

The Museum at Bethel Woods
Sullivan County Historical Society

Books

Dale Bell, ed., *Woodstock: An Inside Look at the Movie that Shook Up the World and Defined a Generation* (Studio City: Michael Wiese, 1999).

Jack Curry, *Woodstock: The Summer of Our Lives* (New York: Weidenfeld & Nicolson, 1989).

John Conway, *Remembering the Sullivan County Catskills* (Charleston: History Press, 2008)

Abbie Hoffman, *Woodstock Nation: A Talk-Rock Album* (New York: Vintage, 1969).

Glen Joshpe, *Joshpe's Journey*, (Stamford: Stonecrest Publishers, 2001).

Lisa Law, *Flashing on the Sixties*, (Santa Rosa: Square Books, 2000).

Joel Makower, *Woodstock: The Oral History* (New York: Doubleday, 1989).

James Perone, *Woodstock: An Encyclopedia f the Music and Art Fair* (Westport: Greenwood Press, 2005).

Joel Rosenman and John Roberts, *Young Men with Unlimited Capital* (New York: Harcourt Brace Jovanovich, 1974).

Bob Spitz, *Barefoot in Babylon: The Creation of the Woodstock Music Festival, 1969* (New York: Norton, 1989).

Elliot Tiber, *Taking Woodstock: A True Story of a Riot, a Concert, and a Life* (Garden City Park, NY: Square One, 2007).

Jean Young and Michael Lang, *Woodstock Festival Remembered* (New York: Ballantine, 1979).

Periodicals

Ellenville *Press* (August 21, 1969).
The Independent (Hillsdale, NY) (July 26, 2002).
Life (August, 1989).
The Medical Post (April 24, 2001).
Middletown, N.Y., *Times Herald-Record* (August 9, 16, 18, 22, 27 1969).
Middletown, N.Y., *Times Herald-Record* (August 12, 1989; March 8, 2006).
Newburgh, N.Y., *Evening Press* (August 21, 1969).
Newsday (August 18, 1969).
New York Sunday News (August 17, 1969).
New York Times (August 18, 19 1969; August 14, 1989; July 1, 2006; May 29, 2008; March 19, 2009).
Port Jervis, N.Y. *Union-Gazette* (August 18, 1969).
Sullivan County Record (Jeffersonville, NY; August 21, 1969).
Sullivan County *Democrat* (Callicoon, N.Y.; August 29, 2006).
Today's Health, July 1970. pp. 20-25, 59-612.
Toronto *Globe & Mail* (August 19, 1969).

Reports

William Abruzzi, M.D., "A White Lake Happening," report to New York State Department of Health, September 2, 1969.

A.F. Cacchillo, Administrator, Community General Hospital, report.

Community General Hospital, Board of Trustees, Business Minutes September 3, 1969.

Community General Hospital, Liberty Diovision, report of admissions August 15-18, 1969.

C.B. Esselstyn, M.D., Director of Emergency Medical Services, New York State Department of Health; report to New York State Department of Health, September 9, 1969.

Food For Love, Inc., "Foodservice Projections for White Lake Music Festival."

Gerald Lieber, P.E., Senior Sanitary Engineer, Monticello Subdistrict; report to New York State Department of Health, September 8, 1969.

Monticello Board of Education, meeting minutes, August 5, 1969 and August 19, 1969.

New York State Department of Health, Albany Regional Office, "Environmental Health and Emergency Medical Services Report on the Woodstock Music and Art Fair (Aquarius Festival), White Lake, Bethel Town, Sullivan County, N.Y., September 25, 1969.

Sydney P. Schiff, M.D., Chief of Staff, Community General Hospital, report.

Norbert Shay, M.D., report to the New York State Department of Health, September 8, 1969.

Woodstock Ventures, "Preliminary Report: Evaluation of Public Health Considerations; New York Department of Health, August 5, 1969

Incidental reports

Sheriff Deputy Harold C Keesler
Sheriff Deputy Phillip Key
Sheriff Deputy Carl Knapp
Sheriff Deputy Jed Reinlies

Sheriff Deputy Michael Rothman
Sheriff Deputy Frank Zurawski
Lt. Ralph Breaky

Interviews

Anna Benson, R.N.
Esther Boddy
Alan Fried, M.D.
A. F. Cacchillo
Martin Cohen
Martin Cowan, M.D.
Gladys Devaney
Alan Fried, M.D.
Gustave Gavis, M.D.
Dennis Glazer, M.D., USAF (Ret.)
Herman Goldfarb, M.D.
Donald Goldmacher, M.D.
Wavy Gravy
Barbara Hahn, R.N.

Liz Hermann, R.N.
Anibel Herrera, M.D.
Lisa Law
Mischa Leshner
Harold Lindsey
Shirley Lowenthal
Jack Maidman, M.D.
Ansel Marks, M.D.
Frances Marks, R.N.
Howard Perlman
Beatrice Pollets, R.N.
Rose Raimond , R.N.
Helen Reno
John Sebastian

Carolyn Sprague
George Spicka
Msg .Edward Straub
R. Peter Uhlmann, M.D.

Al Whittaker
Suzanne White
Seymour Wiener, M.D.
Barbara Wexler, R.N.
Miriam Yasgur

Personal Communications

Ruth Aprilante, R.N.
Michael Baxter, volunteer, Mountaindale FD First Aid Squad
Sam V. Boor, M.D., March 2009
Charles Dombeck
Robert J. Flynn
Harvey Lashinsky
Charles Rudiger, Ph.D.
Lucille Thalmann Rudiger, R.N.
Bryan St. Louis
Albert Sutton, M.D., October 2008

Miscellaneous

Michael Wm. Doyle, Ph.D., Statement on the Historical and Cultural Significance of the 1969 Woodstock Festival Site, September 25, 2001 (http://www.woodstockpreservation.org/SignificanceStatement.htm)

Lisa Law, *Flashing the Sixties: A Tribal Document* (documentary film); Flashback Productions, Ltd. 1994.

Museum at Bethel Woods, Attendees Memories.

Sean McKean, "Beyond the Myth: A deeper look at the 1969 Woodstock Festival," Woodstock Preservation Archives (http://www. woodstockpreservation.org/Essays/BeyondTheMyth.htm)

Office of Vital Records, New York State Department of Health

Woodstock Survival Sheet, accessed March 18, 2009: http://www. geocities.com/Athens/3548/woodstock.html

The Authors

Myron Gittell, RN has worked in the field of health care for more than three decades as a registered nurse and Emergency Medical Technician. He has served as an attendant, driver, and EMT for both volunteer and commercial ambulance services. He is a longtime researcher of the history of emergency care and emergency transportation. His collection of ambulance memorabilia has included four vintage ambulances. He was on the National Advisory Committee of the "To The Rescue" Museum in Roanoke, Virginia, and guest curator of the "Help is Here" Emergency Medical Services history exhibit at the New York State Museum in 2004-2005.

Jack Kelly, EMT is a novelist and writer of nonfiction. He has written about the history of Emergency Medical Services for *American Heritage Magazine* and is the co-author of *EMS Stress.*

Printed in the United States
220779BV00002B/1/P

9 780962 635731